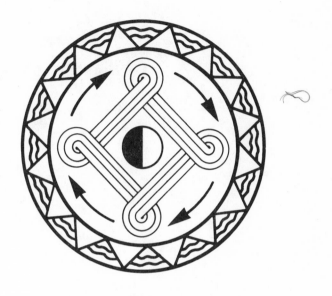

Within and around the ear^th, within and around the hills, within and arc_____ mountains, your authority returns to yo___

# ALTERNATIVE PATHWAYS TO HEALING

*The Recovery
Medicine Wheel*

Kip Coggins, M.S.W.

Health Communications, Inc.
Deerfield Beach, Florida

Library of Congress Cataloging-in-Publication Date

Coggins, Kip
   Alternative pathways to healing: the recovery medicine
wheel/Kip Coggins.
      p.  cm.
   Includes bibliographical references.
   ISBN 1-55874-089-9
   1. Alternative Medicine. 2. Substance Abuse — Alternative Treatment. 3. Indians of North America — Medicine. I. Title.
   R733.C64   1990                                    90-4650
   616.86'06 — dc20                                      CIP

© 1990 Kip Coggins
ISBN 1-55874-089-9

Publisher:  Health Communications, Inc.
                 3201 S.W. 15th Street
                 Deerfield Beach, Florida 33442

Cover design by Ana Bowen

# Dedication

This book is dedicated to Emy S., Cathy M. and Mary H. without whose love, support and assistance this book would never have been made possible.

# Contents

# Introduction

The medicine wheel approach to recovery is a way that can help adult children of alcoholics, co-dependents and chemically dependent persons alike. Individuals who have grown up in a family marked by dysfunction also can derive benefit from walking the steps of the Recovery Medicine Wheel. Although it is based in Native American culture and tradition, the Recovery Medicine Wheel takes a balanced approach to the task of recovery from addiction and addictive ways of living that will appeal to people of diverse cultural backgrounds and spiritual traditions. It has been used successfully at AA (Alcoholics Anonymous) meetings for over a decade.

Within the medicine wheel recovery way, four basic realms of human existence are addressed:

1. The physical realm
2. The realm of knowledge and enlightenment
3. The spiritual realm
4. The realm of introspective thought.

Beyond this, each area of the medicine wheel acts as a complete wheel within that realm.

For example, if you start walking the medicine wheel in the North (physical realm), you will find aspects of the other three directions included therein. This structure gives each section of the wheel a completeness within itself, as well as a connection to the other realms of human existence, the other points on the wheel.

As you walk the steps of the Recovery Medicine Wheel, you often will stop at different points along the way. Perhaps the words will stick in your mind or you may actually see yourself in the wheel. The wheel will act as a mirror for you. At times you will see something that reaffirms you. At other times you may see something in the Recovery Medicine Wheel that will inspire you to make a personal life change. Whatever happens, the intent of the Recovery Medicine Wheel will be the same. It is designed to help you grow healthy mentally, spiritually and physically. It is intended to help you become more fully human, at greater harmony with yourself and achieve inner peace. If used properly, the Recovery Medicine Wheel can help you recover from your dysfunctional past and/or addiction and point you in the direction of greater harmony with your world.

In the chapters ahead, you will grow to understand new ways of thinking and new approaches to living. The means by which you can make positive recovery real for yourself will be presented. The Recovery Medicine Wheel is a path that can lead each and every one of us to greater self-understanding, a path that has the potential of helping us see the truth of addiction. When you know yourself and you can see addiction or any dysfunctional way of living for what it is, the life changes you need to make will become clear. Your desire for healthier, happier living will provide your inspiration. The steps of the Recovery Medicine Wheel will become your tools with which lasting change can be fashioned. Come along with me. Let's recover together.

# 1

# The Beginning Of Awareness

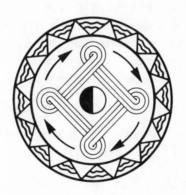

*"Let yourself really hear, really feel, really see. Let yourself be a human being. Only when you are real with yourself can you begin to find the right path in life."*

Tom Lujan/Taos Pueblo/New Mexico, 1988.

### What Is A Medicine Wheel?

The term *medicine*, as it is used in *medicine wheel*, refers to a healing, teaching, enlightening, spiritual energy. A medicine wheel can best be described as a mirror within in which everything is reflected (Storm, 1972).

Books, people, words, flowers, stories and many other entities can be medicine wheels. In fact, any idea, person or object can be a medicine wheel (Storm, 1972). The important thing to understand is that we learn, grow and change by allowing each person, place, object or experience to teach us.

This requires that we expand our ideas of what constitutes learning. If we see our relationship to other people, objects and situations as mirrors to what is going on within our own minds, anything that occurs can carry a lesson for us. Anything can be a medicine wheel.

### What Is The Recovery Medicine Wheel?

The Recovery Medicine Wheel is comprised of the four major realms of human existence:

- *(North)* the physical realm
- *(East)* the realm of knowledge and enlightenment
- *(South)* the spiritual realm
- *(West)* the realm of introspective thought.

Each realm of the Recovery Medicine Wheel has four steps, for a total of 16 when the wheel is considered in its entirety.

Walking the steps of the Recovery Medicine Wheel means choosing a starting point and continuing in a sun-wise direction back to your beginning place (clockwise in the northern hemisphere). Although you can start at any point on the wheel, it seems to work best if you begin with step one in either the West or the North. There is no set limit on the amount of time to be spent working each individual step. Some people may spend a week on a single step, while others may move through the entire circle in that same period of time.

Remember, however, that a circle has no true beginning or ending point. Therefore, competition (as in who can get through the steps of the Recovery Medicine Wheel the fastest) has no meaning. In fact, those who rush through each step in order to get to the next, will find the Recovery Medicine Wheel a much less valuable tool or guide for recovery. When you have worked through all 16 steps and return to your starting point, you are ready to begin again with a new understanding.

## What Makes The Recovery Medicine Wheel Different From Recovery Models Already Being Used?

The Recovery Medicine Wheel is a new path to recovery and growth based on ancient traditions from the first people of North America (North American Indians). Therefore, it is not a fad. Rather, it is an approach to recovery and living employing elements of Native American culture which have been passed down from generation to generation for centuries.

The Recovery Medicine Wheel is a spiritual, emotional, psychological and physical improvement model for those who seek inner peace, spiritual strength and a healthier mind and body. It encourages positive growth and change in all areas of life, and therefore, has the potential of being a powerful tool with which a person can maintain sobriety and sustain recovery.

The Recovery Medicine Wheel is the only step approach in existence that emphasizes a circular as opposed to a linear path to recovery. In this way, it is more in line with the natural movements of the earth, the solar system and the universe. If we stop to think and observe, it becomes clear that seasons move from spring to summer to fall to winter and back to spring. The earth is in a circular orbit around the sun, and the universe moves in cycles wherein planets or stars are born, age and die, only to be born again. So the organization of the Recovery Medicine

Wheel into the directions of the four winds acts as our connection to the natural world.

## How Did The Recovery Medicine Wheel Idea Get Started?

The original idea of this adaption of the Medicine Wheel began about five years ago when I was seeking a meaningful path for my own recovery. In my search, I became acutely aware that no recovery format existed which took into account my entire being, including my Native American culturally based spirituality. I felt the need for something more in recovery, something that would address the whole person. With this in mind, I began working on a step approach that touches on all aspects of life: physical, psychological, spiritual and emotional. In addition, I designed this approach to be culturally and spiritually sensitive to the needs of Native American and natural people.

In the summer of 1987, the Recovery Medicine Wheel was officially put on paper. I thought it would be of use only to Native Americans or those with a similar spiritual and cultural orientation. What I found, however, was that many people were able to relate to the concepts found in the Recovery Medicine Wheel, even those who were not at all familiar with Native American spirituality. Many adult children of alcoholics, co-dependent and chemically dependent persons from diverse backgrounds seemed interested in the Recovery Medicine Wheel approach. It was at that point I began to realize the potential the Recovery Medicine Wheel had of becoming a viable, alternative path to recovery for large numbers of people.

## What Is An ACoA?

An ACoA is an Adult Child of an Alcoholic. This term is used to refer to any person who grew up in a home where the adult caregiver or caregivers (usually, but not always parents) were, or continue to be, alcoholic. However, people can have the characteristics of ACoAs if their parents were not even alcoholic at all. This occurs when the parents or caregivers are themselves adult children of alcoholics and have continued to mimic the dysfunctional patterns of interaction they learned in their own families of origin (Kritsberg, 1986).

Some of the more common characteristics of adult children of alcoholics (Woititz, 1985) are listed below:

## ACoA Characteristics

1. ACoAs have problems with trust.
2. ACoAs often feel incompetent and fear others will find out.
3. ACoAs have difficulty handling change.
4. ACoAs are extremely self-critical.
5. ACoAs often have a sense of impending doom.
6. ACoAs constantly fear failure.
7. ACoAs generally have a low sense of self-worth.
8. ACoAs often harbor a great deal of anger and resentment toward their alcoholic parent(s), coupled with a sense of guilt for having these feelings.
9. ACoAs often feel a great deal of shame over what has occurred in their families.
10. ACoAs tend to become discouraged easily.

Additional characteristics of ACoAs include the following:

### *An Inability To Accept Positive Feedback From Others*

When confronted with a compliment or a commendation, ACoAs will downplay or minimize. They have trouble seeing themselves in a positive light and, therefore, find it hard to accept praise from others.

### *Difficulty Seeing Themselves As Capable Persons*

ACoAs are survivors yet often are unable to recognize this quality in themselves. They generally perceive their achievements in life as luck, a fluke or a mistake. Statements such as, "I guess I was just in the right place at the right time," are common.

## *Internal Emptiness*

In general ACoAs feel empty inside. This emptiness is like an emotional spiritual hole that leaves them feeling incomplete. As a result, most ACoAs feel they don't quite measure up, that they are somehow flawed.

## *Manipulation And People-Pleasing As A Means Of Survival*

ACoAs have a fear of being themselves, of letting their real feelings be known. They tend to believe they have to win the support of friends, co-workers, bosses, etc., so they engage in manipulative people-pleasing behavior designed to get others to like them. The problem with this way of living is that it leaves ACoAs with a constant feeling of fear; fear of being "found out," of being discovered for who and what they really are. And what do ACoAs believe they are? Incompetent, unlovable and bad are just a few words that describe how they feel about themselves. This negativity in self-view is the emotional baggage ACoAs carry with them from their families of origin right into adult life.

## What Is A Co-dependent?

Simply stated, co-dependency is a disease in much the same way as chemical dependency. Co-dependence grows out of the disease process known as addiction (Schaef, 1986). It is often the spouse of an addicted person who is identified as co-dependent. However, this is not always the case. Children, parents and even friends of the addicted person can become co-dependent.

The co-dependent person is often the one who is closest emotionally to the chemically dependent individual. He or she becomes focused on stopping the addiction in that person. As attempts to stop the addicted person from continuing with chemical use fail, the co-dependent person tries harder, becomes more depressed and desperate, focusing even more intensely on the addiction of the chemically dependent person.

Although co-dependent people will exhibit a number of different behaviors and symptoms, there are commonalities.

## Co-dependent Characteristics

Listed below are some of the characteristics more frequently observed (Schaef, 1986) in or manifested by co-dependents:

### *Issues Of Control*

Co-dependents try desperately to control situations. They attempt to manage the lives of everyone around them, especially the person with the chemical addiction.

### *Caretaking*

Co-dependents often fear that their only real worth in life is in what they can do for others. Therefore, they become very involved in "taking care of," which gives them their main sense of place and purpose.

### *Martyrdom*

Co-dependents will endure suffering for the purpose of saving a marriage, keeping the family together or keeping the chemically addicted person from harm or shame. In the process they are actually perpetuating the problem by making excuses for, cleaning up after and putting up with the behaviors of the addicted person upon whom all attention has been focused.

### *Being Out Of Touch With Feelings*

Co-dependents tend to be so preoccupied with the feelings and concerns of others that they deny their own. They will often allow themselves to have only acceptable or good feelings. Co-dependents deny or repress feelings of anger and resentment. As co-dependents deny their own needs to be nurtured, they become depressed, possessive and jealous.

## What Are Chemically Addicted People Like?

First and foremost, chemically addicted people are suffering from a disease process in which they are physically and/or psychologically dependent on a chemical substance, be it alcohol or some other drug. In this book, the terms chemically dependent, drug addicted, alcohol addicted, chemically addicted and simply addicted are used interchangeably. The reason for this is one of familiarizing you with the different terms used in the field of chemical dependence or substance abuse treatment and recovery. In addition, the constant interchange of terms is designed to encourage you to think of addiction and addictive processes in broader terms.

As you will discover in this book and in life, addiction is not limited to chemical substances. People can become addicted to work, activities, lifestyles, family roles and even other people. In each of these cases an addictive approach to life and living is in place. Therefore, the focus in treatment and recovery needs to be on growing beyond addictive life patterns. If this is not accomplished, the addicted person runs the risk of simply moving from one addiction to another with very little real change in his or her approach to living.

Below are some of the traits commonly found among addicted people. Again these traits are not to be thought of as being characteristic of only those persons who are addicted to a chemical substance, i.e., alcohol. Rather, these characteristics are to be thought of as being common to the addictive process, whether manifested in the form of alcoholism, workaholism, drug dependence, compulsive consumption of food or what have you.

## Addictive Characteristics

### Compulsive Thinking And Behavior

Addicted people will constantly seek out, consume or think of that person, place or thing upon which they have become focused. This compulsion can and does take on a quality of urgency and obsession which seems to totally consume, dominate or control all areas of the addicted person's life.

## Self-Delusion

Addicted people will lie to and attempt to manipulate everyone around them, themselves included. They often will make such statements as, "I don't have to worry, I can stop any time."

## Rationalization

Addicted people will make statements such as, "I have to drink at weddings because it would be socially unacceptable not to." Or "I can't be alcoholic because I never drink before 5:00 p.m." or "If you want to see a real drug addict, look at a junkie, now that's a drug addict" or even "Sure, I use coke, but doesn't everybody?"

## Intellectualization

Addicted people are able to discuss at length the seriousness of another person's drugging or drinking behavior. They can even talk about the risks of overworking, overeating or overdoing in any area of life. However, when it comes time to discuss him or herself, the addicted person will simply fail to see that she or he has a problem.

## Feelings Of (Or Fear Of) Rejection

Addicted people often feel they are unloved, unwanted and of little worth. This is why they develop addictive behaviors. Addiction helps them avoid feelings. To feel is far too fearful, too painful, so they take solace in whatever makes them feel good, be it drugs, food, relationships, work, alcohol or whatever.

## Pseudo Or False Independence

Addicted people often will exhibit a pseudo-independent exterior, while inside they long to be cared for, nurtured and loved. They will characterize themselves as stoic persons, as loners. This projection of a tough exterior is often used by the addicted person to maintain emotional distance from others, as well as from her or himself.

In addition to the characteristics already listed, addicted persons (Forrest, 1981), also exhibit or experience:

1. Anxiety                    6. Self-centeredness
2. Anger                      7. Impatience
3. Manipulative Behavior      8. Irresponsibility
4. Denial                     9. Immaturity
5. Depression

Certainly, there will be those who question whether or not the characteristics listed above apply to their particular addiction or to the addictions of other persons.

For example, most people would not consider a workaholic to be irresponsible or in denial. However, if we take a closer look, we may find the workaholic denies health problems by refusing to exercise, eat properly or monitor his or her blood pressure. She or he may be very responsible at work but very irresponsible at home, i.e., not keeping promises made to children, not working at maintaining a healthy marriage. In the final analysis, the underlying life dynamics of the workaholic are the same as those of other addicted persons. Just like the alcoholic, the workaholic has a single activity (work) which has become so central in her or his life that important areas of physical and emotional health have been compromised.

So you see, conceiving of addiction as being manifested by chemical dependency alone is far too narrow a view of this broad-reaching disease process. This disease (addiction) can destroy lives both emotionally and physically. Those who suffer include not only the addicted person, but family members, spouses and friends.

As you read keep in mind that addiction does not exist in individuals in isolation. It is not only a result of alcohol, cocaine or heroin. Rather, addiction is a result of addictive approaches to life, and these life patterns can be found throughout our modern society. We work, recreate, exercise, love and, in general, live addictively. Therefore, whether we are ACoA, co-dependent, chemically dependent or simply addicted to some person, place or thing, we are all touched by this disease.

Now is the time for us to stop playing those addictive games of blaming, comparing and trying to live safely within our self-righteousness. It is time for us to understand and acknowledge that regardless of how we manifest or are touched by addiction, the underlying feelings of anger, guilt, depression and low self-esteem are the same. Therefore, let us begin to walk the path of greater knowledge of ourselves and others. Let us heal ourselves together in the Recovery Medicine Wheel way.

# 2

# Walking
# The Steps

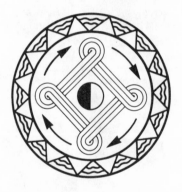

*"The teachings of our grandfathers are everywhere around us, but it is up to each of us to seek out that knowledge."*

*Harry Yazzie/Navajo/New Mexico, 1989.*

## NORTH
### (Physical Realm)

1. Take good physical care of myself.
2. Regain balance in my life by developing an understanding of the important connection between the physical, psychological, spiritual and emotional parts of my existence.
3. Stop inflicting pain (either physical or emotionally) on others or myself.
4. Come to an understanding that change is a process. (I can't expect miracles overnight.)

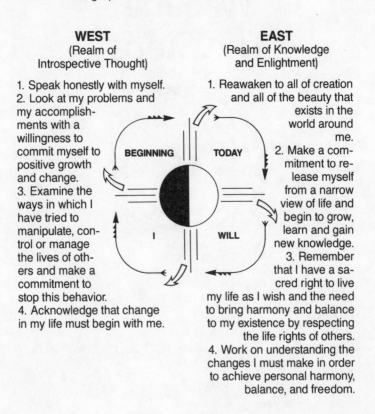

## WEST
### (Realm of Introspective Thought)

1. Speak honestly with myself.
2. Look at my problems and my accomplishments with a willingness to commit myself to positive growth and change.
3. Examine the ways in which I have tried to manipulate, control or manage the lives of others and make a commitment to stop this behavior.
4. Acknowledge that change in my life must begin with me.

## EAST
### (Realm of Knowledge and Enlightment)

1. Reawaken to all of creation and all of the beauty that exists in the world around me.
2. Make a commitment to release myself from a narrow view of life and begin to grow, learn and gain new knowledge.
3. Remember that I have a sacred right to live my life as I wish and the need to bring harmony and balance to my existence by respecting the life rights of others.
4. Work on understanding the changes I must make in order to achieve personal harmony, balance, and freedom.

## SOUTH
### (Spiritual Realm)

1. Come to an understanding of my special relation to Mother Earth. (Release my pain to Mother Earth).
2. Come to an understanding of my special relation to Father Sky.
3. Seek a greater understanding of my sacred connection to all of the Universe.
4. Reconnect with and nurture my own Spirit.

This is the Recovery Medicine Wheel. The individual steps are guides for those who seek spiritual, emotional, psychological and physical growth or improvement. In this section, a brief description of each step will be given. The reason for brevity is one of allowing you, the reader, an opportunity to gain a basic understanding of the Recovery Medicine Wheel, while at the same time encouraging you to search for your own answers, to look for the meaning of each step in your life.

While reading through the descriptions of each step, try to keep an open mind. Hold your opinions, judgments and explorations until after you have completed the entire chapter. This will give you the chance to experience the Recovery Medicine Wheel in totality.

As you return to certain steps for further investigation or contemplation, remember that those steps which intrigue, inspire or disturb you most are the same steps that hold important clues to your own recovery.

Why is this so? Because our reactions to persons, places, events and ideas are mirrors for what is going on inside ourselves.

For example, if the Recovery Medicine Wheel step that addresses manipulation makes you feel angry or uneasy, perhaps it is because you, yourself, are a manipulative person or have allowed yourself to be manipulated by others. On the other hand, if you are inspired by the step that asks you to commit yourself to positive growth and change, it is likely that you have reached a point in your life where change is desired and the Recovery Medicine Wheel is merely acting as a catalyst.

Remember, however, that this medicine wheel, these steps, are only tools for you in the process of recovery. They cannot recover for you.

Think of these steps as you would the paddle of a canoe. The paddle has great potential for moving you along the river. But it is up to you to put the paddle in the water, push forward and adjust to the current. In the same way the steps of the Recovery Medicine Wheel have great potential for moving you along in the river of life and recovery. But you must use them. You must apply them sincerely. Otherwise, they will be no more than words . . . black scratches on a paper.

## The Steps

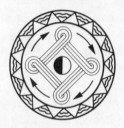

### *North: The Physical Realm*

The North is the physical realm of the world. In the North heavy snows fall each year. When spring comes, after the long cold winter has purified the land, trees and flowers burst into bloom, waters run clear and cold, animals awaken from their long sleep, frogs sing and the warm winds whisper. Spring in the North is a time of sudden rebirth after a long period of cold silence. We will begin here because it is a time of rebirth. You have made a decision in your life to stop physically abusing your body. You have come out of a long sleep. You are now ready for rebirth.

### Step 1: Beginning Today I Will Take Good Physical Care Of Myself

This first step is simple, but the meaning extends into many areas of life and applies to many people. If you are abusing drugs or alcohol, this step applies to you. It means that to begin walking through the medicine wheel of recovery, you must start by recognizing the damage you are inflicting on your body through the use of drugs or alcohol.

If you are an adult child of an alcoholic or a co-dependent person, this step means you need to look at your own physical health. You need to ask yourself whether or not you have neglected your own physical needs. You may be eating poorly, not getting the exercise you need or simply not getting a break from the stresses of your life with a drug or alcohol dependent person.

This first step means that starting today you will begin to make the changes you need to bring about improved physical health. If you are eating a poorly balanced diet, you must change that. If you are not getting the release from stress or the exercise you require, you need to arrange your day to allow for both physical activity and relaxation. If you are abusing drugs or alcohol, you must stop. If you are addicted to any substance, lifestyle or person, you must get treatment for that addiction. Your treatment will depend on your current problem and the severity of that problem.

For example, you may need inpatient care at a chemical dependency unit to help you overcome physical addiction. If so, this will be your first step in taking good physical care of yourself. If you are addicted to a person or lifestyle, getting outpatient treatment may be *your* first step. Whatever the path, the first step in recovery must lead you in the direction of taking better physical care of yourself.

### Step 2: Beginning Today I Will Regain Balance In My Life By Developing An Understanding Of The Important Connection Between The Physical, Psychological, Spiritual And Emotional Parts Of My Existence

This means you will begin to see the entire picture of your life. For example, if a person simply moves away from his or her dysfunctional family, only one life dynamic has been changed. That same person may continue to feel fear, confusion, loneliness and a sense of not belonging. That is because he or she has only changed one part of his or her existence. To start on the path of recovery, that same person must begin to look at emotions, moods, self-perception, sense of meaning in life and so forth. The following may clarify step two:

Understanding the wholeness of life is like understanding a tree. If one looks at a leaf alone or at a piece of root, one will understand only that part of the tree. But if one steps back and looks at the entire tree, it becomes much easier to see how all the parts of the tree connect to one another. So it is with life. If one looks at only a single part of life, the total meaning becomes lost, obscured. Therefore, when one considers life, it is wise to step back and view the many different parts. In this way one can understand how experiences, feelings, health and dreams connect to and affect one another.

What this passage is saying is that you will need to start monitoring your feelings (your highs and lows). Look carefully at what causes emotional distress for you. In addition, look at how this stress affects the way you feel and behave.

- Do you get stomach aches when you are nervous?
- Do you give up on your health resolutions when you are depressed?
- Does your life dream flicker or die when you meet with failure or setbacks?
- How does it affect you physically?
- How do all of your behaviors, experiences and feelings impact on your physical well-being?
- How does your physical health affect you emotionally, psychologically and spiritually?

In other words, this step is asking you to understand that physical well-being involves the need to become enlightened, to become aware of the important connection between emotions, life stress, sense of self and the effect all these life elements have on your physical health.

### Step 3: Beginning Today I Will Stop Inflicting Pain (Either Physical Or Emotional) On Others Or Myself

At this point on the medicine wheel we need to look at the pain we are inflicting on others and on ourselves. This pain can be displayed in many forms. Perhaps you are a person who drinks too much and becomes violent. It could be that you have physically or sexually abused your child or another person while intoxicated. If you have not actually physically touched another person, you may have inflicted emotional pain on others with hurtful or hateful words.

You may be very angry if you live with an addicted person, or even if you have moved away from that person. By displaying your anger to that person, you are inflicting pain. Yes, you must release your anger but, no, you must not do it by inflicting pain. If you are lashing out at a spouse, a sibling, a child, a parent, a partner or a friend, you are inflicting pain. If you hurt inside, if you have anger or pain within you, you must release it at a safe time and in a safe manner. The ways in which anger and pain can be released will be explained later. For the moment, however, all you need to know is that you must stop inflicting pain. The pain you inflict on others eventually damages you, and the pain you inflict on yourself (which includes abuse of drugs or alcohol) eventually will damage others as well. Therefore, look at the pain in your life. If you are causing pain in any form, it must stop . . . beginning today.

## Step 4: Beginning Today I Will Come To An Understanding That Change Is A Process (I Can't Expect Miracles Overnight)

For those recovering from an addiction, this step is very difficult. Recovering addicts are used to immediate gratification and the thought of going through a process can seem unfamiliar, even frightening. Adult children of alcoholics and/or dysfunctional families also will be distressed by this step. Most recovering adult children who go to a therapist to find out what is wrong want to be better right now! They often can see the ideal or goal of health and integration they desire, but at the same time, they feel incapable of going through the process needed to achieve that goal. This is actually not all that hard to understand. After all, adult children of alcoholics are from families where seeking instant gratification was the common mode of behavior.

In general, people from dysfunctional families are not accustomed to process living. Dysfunctional families go from crisis to crisis with little time or space left for problem resolution. Children in these families are seldom aware of the causes of anger or distress in their parents and since no formula exists for resolving a problem, no one can ever reasonably predict an outcome. Therefore, recovering people must *learn* to live life as a process. As the following explains:

> You cannot plant a field of corn in the morning and expect a crop by nightfall. The corn must be hoed, watered and tended throughout the summer. By season's end, the gardener's careful attention will result in a beautiful crop.

So it is with the process of recovery. Time and work will result in a positive change. But just as corn is beautiful from kernel to crop, so is your growth in the process of recovery.

Understand that change takes time. You can't expect miracles overnight, but you can expect miracles over time.

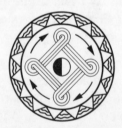

### East: The Realm Of Knowledge And Enlightenment

The East is the realm of knowledge and enlightenment. Each day when the sun rises in the East, it sheds light on all the land. The East is the morning direction. It is the direction of new day, new light, new thought and new resolve. The East is the realm within where we expand our views, learn new ways and rediscover forgotten zest in living.

I remember a time when I was much younger. Our family lived near the forest. On summer mornings the birds would loudly greet the day as the sun broke over the horizon far out in Lake Huron. I recall the joy I felt as I looked out at all creation. I would wonder, what will I do today? What will I find? The world was so very beautiful and the beauty filled me with a sense of excited curiosity of what the day might bring. Mornings are still very special for me. Each day I see the new light as a chance to make positive changes, to continue growing and learning. I still see mornings as a time of great beauty, a time when I am filled with that sense of excited inquisitiveness.

### Step 1: Beginning Today I Will Reawaken To All Creation And All Of The Beauty That Exists In The World Around Me

This step is an important beginning for those who seek recovery. A close friend of mine who uses the Recovery Medicine Wheel daily states, "My own recovery didn't really get under way until I reawakened to the beauty of the creation around me. After years of being a family caretaker and going through my own struggle with addiction, I had shut myself off from much of the world around me. For nearly five years I stopped collecting herbal medicinal plants in the forest, I stopped watching the changes of Lake Michigan across the road from my house; I missed many sunrises and sunsets. I also stopped being open to new people and new knowledge. The result was that I became an isolated, angry and depressed person. Finally, I realized that my own recovery and growth would never get fully underway until I opened myself up again.

"Now when I look at the hills or mountains or lake, I really see and feel the wonder of creation. But just saying, 'Okay, I'm ready to be open,' doesn't do the trick.

"Like everything worthwhile, opening up again takes work. I went to groups, talked with a counselor and drummed and meditated for many months. Finally, on a cold, clear night in late winter, I stopped my car on a deserted gravel road. I had often driven down that road in the past to be alone with nature and to meditate. This time I put some tobacco on the earth and started to use my drum. When I looked up at the stars, an almost electric energy filled my soul. I began to cry. The tears came not from a place of sorrow, but from a place of healing. That very moment was the reopening of my heart. It was my reawakening to all of creation."

This step means that you as a recovering person must learn again to see the world around you. Perhaps you shut off your awareness of that world because it seemed only ugly and painful. But in shutting out the pain, you also closed the door to beauty, positivity and the awesomeness of creation. In this step you must again open your eyes, ears and other senses. Feel the beauty of a breeze. Cherish the smell of a flower. Become excited by a sunrise or a bird's song. Learn to see the beauty in other people. In essence, begin to *be* again. Open yourself up to new experiences, new persons and new awareness. Leave behind the chemicals and concepts that hinder your growth and development as a human being. Begin today to be, to become, to live.

## Step 2: Beginning Today I Will Release Myself From A Narrow View Of Life And Begin To Grow, Learn And Gain New Knowledge

In this second step, you must begin to give up your narrow and often self-destructive view of life. Perhaps you have closed yourself off from new experiences because your addiction (or the addiction of another person) has somehow forced you into a rigid family role or self-view that you feel incapable of transcending. Perhaps you were abused as a child and feel you are not worthy of any more respect or consideration in life than you already have. Whatever the case, this step challenges you to venture forth. In this step, you are called upon to learn, grow and gain new knowledge.

At this point on the medicine wheel, you need to open yourself up to new paths of learning, new ways of understanding and new ways of viewing yourself. Growth beyond a narrow view of life means understanding addiction in yourself or another, as well as developing new ways of solving problems, coping with change, dealing with stress and learning to have a life dream again. In this step you will learn to go beyond your fear, to begin feeling and believing that you are worthwhile, that you can make a positive life change.

### Step 3: Beginning Today I Will Remember That I Have A Sacred Right To Live My Life As I Wish And The Need To Bring Harmony And Balance To My Existence By Respecting The Life Rights Of Others

What this step means is that you have a right to be you. You do not have to play the role assigned you by your dysfunctional family. In fact, you need to be freed from the rigid roles in order to grow. If you are co-dependent, you must let go of that other person's addiction. If you are a recovering addict, you must let family members and friends know that you no longer choose to use alcohol and drugs and that by making that choice you are exercising your rights.

However, as step three states, you must also respect the life rights of others. This means that you need to be ever mindful of the fine line between your expression of self and the boundaries of another person's existential rights.

For example, if you are an adult child of an alcoholic, you have a right to your anger and resentment and a need to work through it. Nevertheless, you also must remember that working through your anger by lashing out at your actively alcoholic or recovering parent is disrespectful of that person's life rights. Attacking a person with hateful or hurtful words is a form of emotional pain and is therefore disrespectful. To inflict pain on another is disrespectful of that person's sacred existence.

Likewise, a parent who insists (for whatever reason) that an adult child abandon her or his life dream also is being disrespectful of that person's sacred existence. An example of this form of disrespect is a parent who insists that her adult child stay home to care for her. This parent may not insist outright but instead induces guilt, fear or dependency to keep that person from becoming a complete adult.

The Ojibwa Indian story of original man and the fire-keeper's daughter tells us:

> Their responsibility was to care for their children and prepare them for the work of the Creator. They were never to feel that they owned their children, or that the work or desires of their children should be the same as their own. Firekeeper's Daughter remembered the ache in her heart when she saw her children leave their home to go to each of the four directions. However, she was also happy and proud that her children represented the beginnings of the first people of the earth. (Benton-Banai, 1979).

Here we are given an example of a healthy functional family in which the parents allow their children to grow and leave the system. Yes, they care for their children, but they do not force them into predetermined rigid roles through guilt or coercion.

This passage shows us that growing and separating bring necessary grief to be processed as a natural part of growth and change. Firekeeper's Daughter is able to take pride in her children, the paths they have chosen and the people they are becoming. She does not beg her children to stay. She does not sabotage their attempts to establish themselves outside of the family system. In short, she allows them to become fully human, fully adult. She does not stop loving her children and they do not stop loving her. Firekeeper's Daughter simply realizes that her children must become complete people — people who as adults will love her, but also will have their own lives.

Beyond our families, we need to have love and respect for others as well. All caring and concern is not co-dependence. There must be a part within each of us that cares for others, that has compassion.

The real task becomes one of loving ourselves and others. Always putting ourselves ahead of others, regardless of the circumstances, is selfishness. Always putting the needs of others ahead of our own needs is co-dependence. Therefore, our sacred right to live our lives as we wish must be a balance. Just as we must learn how to take charge in our own lives, we also must learn when and where our expression of self, or our desire to have things as we wish, may be infringing upon the rights of others. As we balance our rights, needs and desires with those of others, we will achieve a harmony that will allow us to grow and become fully human.

### Step 4: Beginning Today I Will Work On Understanding The Changes I Must Make In Order To Achieve Personal Harmony, Balance And Freedom

Whereas the previous step emphasized balance in the recognition of life rights of ourselves and others, this step is more personal. It speaks of the changes that must occur within. This step is meant to encourage you to review what may have been learned in the previous steps and take action.

For example, if you remain in a co-dependent role with your spouse, you must develop a plan to break out of this role. If you do not know how to break from a behavioral pattern, this is the point at which you can begin the learning that will lead to positive change. Perhaps you do not feel strong enough to detach from a person, role or relationship alone. In that case, you need to seek out a support group to help you through the process.

If you are a chemically dependent person, you must begin to understand the changes that will help you achieve personal harmony, balance and freedom. This means you need to go beyond simply removing drugs and alcohol from your life to considering the cognitive and behavioral changes that will bring you freedom from addiction. The way you think or view yourself is very important. Your thinking (cognition) can either set you up for relapse into active addiction or free you. For example, you will have a much harder time staying drug-free if you think you never will be able to resist drugs. Likewise, if you behave in an addictive manner in any area of your life, i.e., eating, working, smoking or if you never explore new avenues of thought, new lifestyles or new situations, you never will have the opportunity to acquire different problem-solving skills or coping mechanisms. Your basic approach to life, therefore, will not have changed and you will be more likely to either relapse or move on to a new addiction.

The changes made here must move us away from old, dysfunctional, destructive life patterns to new, balanced, functional ways of living. This means that families or people who discourage expression of feelings must start being more open. Fear must be replaced with a feeling of personal strength through the caring support of the self by the self and of the self by others. Cooperation must replace tyrannical control and love must replace self-hatred.

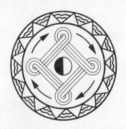

## South: The Spiritual Realm

When the wind blows from the South, a sense of timelessness is felt. When the South is thought of, visions of warmth, comfort and closeness to the earth are conjured up. On the occasions when I have meditated on, contemplated and communed with the South direction, I have felt an incredibly peaceful connection with the earth, the sky, the universe and the beauty of my own existence.

The South is the realm of existence where we will make a connection with a spiritual power greater than ourselves. Some may see this greater power as the collective essence of all people. Others may think of this higher power as the Great Spirit or God, while still others may see this power as being pure energy. It does not matter how a person conceives of her or his higher power and it does not matter if each of us has a different idea of what that higher power is. What does matter is that every recovering person connects with a spiritual essence, a power that is greater than him or herself.

## Step 1: Beginning Today I Will Come To An Understanding Of My Special Relation To Mother Earth (Release My Pain To Mother Earth)

In this step we see the earth as the mother of all living things. We come to realize the earth herself is a living being. In becoming aware of our relationship to Mother Earth, we also begin to understand the healing qualities that lie therein.

With her soil, the earth can nurture us by bringing forth plants as food for us and other living creatures. The stone, soil or trees that are in, of or on the earth can give us shelter. If we know and respect the earth, she will always provide for us. We are not as close to or connected with the earth as we once were . . . which is why all of us must reconnect now with our Mother Earth. We need to take time now to marvel at the large mountain and the small round pebble.

The earth will play a very important role in your own recovery. The earth will heal you with her energy and beauty. She will reaffirm you, as you understand your right to exist is equal to every other living thing. Mother Earth will never reject you or demean you in any way. She is eternally there for you if you will only reach out and touch her.

Let the earth heal you. Touch Mother Earth and ask her to remove your inner sadness, anxiety and fear. Ask Mother Earth to help you let go of the emotional distress that is blocking your recovery and keeping you from breaking the cycle of negative thinking and negative self-perception. Release your pain to Mother Earth and you will be rejuvenated, released, reborn and freed.

## Step 2: Beginning Today I Will Come To An Understanding Of My Special Relation To Father Sky

Father Sky is wind, rain, snow, thunder and lightning, stillness, movement, clarity and cloudiness. Father Sky can be both life-giving and life-taking, tender and terrible.

From Father Sky (the male entity) comes the seeds of rain that nourish the womb of our Mother Earth. However, tornadoes, hurricanes and violent storms come from the sky as well. So how are we to correlate this combination of tenderness and fury? When we watch the sky, we see there is a balance between opposing forces over time and over the face of the earth. Within this balanced way the sky is in harmony.

This teaches us that we, too, must have balance between the opposing forces within our spirits, minds and bodies. All the moods and movements displayed by Father Sky live within each of us as human beings here on earth. We cannot live in a balanced way if we only allow ourselves to be all gentleness or all storm. We must learn to experience and express both the caring and the anger that exist within each of us.

We must keep in mind that when we express anger, we need to do it at a safe time, in a safe place and in a safe manner. We must not harm others physically or emotionally in the process. In order for balance to be maintained, anger must be recognized and released. Likewise, we need to learn not to crush feelings of tenderness. When we want to be loving or caring or quiet or mild in our manner, we need to allow ourselves to do so. Gentleness, too, must have recognition and a means by which it can be expressed.

Beyond this, the sky also teaches us how to protect our spirits from harm. Harmful and destructive people are like the winds of great storms. When those storms occur, we need to take shelter in a safe place. We need to protect ourselves. In the same way, gentleness from other people can be like calmness and sunshine. At those times and with those people, we can become more carefree, open and sharing.

In your recovery the sky will be a mirror for you, reflecting the many moods of humankind. Father Sky will act as a reminder of the feelings within you (both gentle and destructive). If you watch and respect the ways of Father Sky, you will understand the meaning of balance and feel within you a sense of strength and ability. You will know the energizing connection between yourself and the sky as you touch the wind and become one with its movement. As you consciously breathe in life-giving air, you will be filled with awareness; you will grow to understand the connection between yourself and creation.

**Step 3: Beginning Today I Will Seek A Greater Understanding Of My Sacred Connection To All Of The Universe**

This step teaches us to understand humility and belonging. If we contemplate the entire universe, knowing that it extends into infinity, we cannot help but feel humbled. In our humility we have a sense of awe and wonder at being part of this complete yet never-ending totality. We recall that the universe includes everything. In essence, the universe is both creator and creation. Each of us has within ourselves a piece of that universal energy, the same universal energy that is within all other living creatures, stones, water, wind, sun, moon and on and on. This is our connection. We all spring from the same energy source, an energy source that is given to all. It is our choice what we do with our universal energy, which is the common bond between ourselves, our best friends and our worst enemies.

In recovery we can use this common bond, this universal connectedness, to provide support for others who are recovering. We can continue to heal ourselves by sharing knowledge and love with others. However, this love and connectedness must be supportive and uplifting. It must be given freely with no expectation of particular outcome or desire for reciprocation.

It should not be the kind of love you expected in the past or had expected of you when alcohol or drugs were involved. That type of love is not love at all. It is a cry to have emptiness filled. But that emptiness cannot be filled by anyone or anything because that empty person, whether you or someone else, has no self-love. That person is like a bucket with no bottom. All the water in the world will not fill that bucket. Until that person says, "I am going to begin caring for myself, and accept the love and support of others," no amount of love and support will make any difference. However, when that person realizes her or his sacred place in the universe, love and support will act as rain on springtime soil and beautiful things will begin to grow.

### Step 4: Beginning Today I Will Reconnect With And Nuture My Own Spirit

This is perhaps the most direct yet difficult step within the spiritual realm. Within all other spiritual steps, you may have been able to discuss or even philosophize about your spirituality and your connectedness to earth, sky and universe. This step is different. It asks you to nurture your own spirit. To do this, you must connect with your inner self, with that most private part of you. You must be able to acknowledge your fears, desires, emotions and feelings of distress. Most of all, you must learn how to care for your own spirit.

Think of your spirit as a child. Has this child been alone, crying, in need of care? Find out what can be done to help that child. See if the child needs love, reassurance or comforting.

Is that child angry? If so, perhaps you need to let that child express some anger. Find a safe time and place for that child to let the anger go. That safe time and place may be in a therapist's office, in a support group or in the solitude of your own room. The important thing is to let that anger go. Find a place, find a way and let your spirit (your angry child) release that emotion.

If your spirit is in pain from loneliness or being hurt by others, you need to find a path to healing. Just as a crying child is healed by the comfort of a loving, giving mother, your spirit needs to be cared for. Perhaps you will under-stand better what must be done if you again think of your spirit as a child. If that child needs comforting and healing, you may need to touch the earth, let the pain be removed and in the process help your spirit/child be healed. If your spirit/child is lonely, you may need to speak with him or her more often.

If you cannot reach your spirit/child alone, seek the help of another person. You should find someone who will be caring, supportive and nonjudgmental. For if you seek the help of noncaring, negative people, your spirit/child will become even more remote and difficult to find. Treat your spirit, yourself, with love. Seek out your inner self. Reconnect with and nurture that inner self. Heal your spirit.

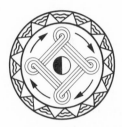

## West: The Realm Of Introspective Thought

West is the sunset direction. The West has elements of both completion and transformation within its realm. At sunset, the day is coming to an end. The day is transforming, changing into night. Just as day transforms to night, our thoughts need to change from an outward direction to an inward one. The West is the realm of introspection and reflection.

Whenever I have meditated on the westward direction, I have become aware of many truths about myself. Some truths have been recognition of my accomplishments that day or in my life to this point. Other truths have been acknowledgment of my own problems, concerns, fears and so on. The western realm has been, and continues to be, a very important part of the medicine wheel for me. It is a realm in which I can acknowledge my accomplishments, review my problems and gather the self-knowledge that will help me make positive life changes. The realm of introspective thought, the West, is the realm within which we must begin to look inside ourselves and be honest with what we see or find.

## Step 1: Beginning Today I Will Speak Honestly With Myself

This step is very straightforward and appears simple. Nevertheless many people, including perhaps yourself, have great difficulty with self-honesty. You may have hidden fears, anger or desires that you have suppressed for so long that accessing those feelings is foreign and even frightening. If you are addicted to a chemical substance, a lifestyle or a person, this step is asking you to acknowledge that addiction, as well as to be honest about other problems in your life. This step is asking you to stop suppressing feelings, stop turning off emotions and stop denying that problems exist.

For example, if you are an adult child of an alcoholic, you may want to appear helpful, calm and in control. However, your reality is that you may be acting helpful as a means of avoiding rejection. You may be displaying calmness as a way of hiding inner tension and fear. Your controlled exterior is likely an attempt to cover up your feelings of failure and inadequacy. To be healed through the medicine wheel, you will need to begin speaking honestly with yourself. You must access those hidden feelings, fears and suppressed emotions. As you explore and acknowledge the truths of your current life experiences, the path to recovery . . . the choices you must make . . . will become clear.

## Step 2: Beginning Today I Will Look At My Problems And My Accomplishments With A Willingness To Commit Myself To Positive Growth And Change

This step may sound like an inventory of positive and negative, but it is much more than that. A person's ability to look at both problems and accomplishments can be an indicator of her or his sense of self. Someone who sees only problems or personal shortcomings might still be punishing her or himself for some failure in life, either real or imagined. Conversely, a person who speaks only of accomplishments is often attempting to convince self and others that no problems exist, that she or he has everything under control. When used properly, however, this step can help the recovering person gain a more balanced sense of self.

For example, if you are a mother who is addicted to drugs or alcohol, you need to acknowledge that addiction as a problem. If you also have provided for your children in spite of difficult circumstances, you must learn to see this as an accomplishment. Furthermore, when you make the decision to remove drugs and alcohol from your life, while also deciding to repair whatever damage the relationship with your children has sustained in the process, you will have committed yourself to positive growth and change.

If you are an adult child of an alcohol- or drug-addicted parent, you may feel that you have failed at stopping your parent's addiction. As a result you might be viewing yourself as incapable in many areas of life. This negative self-view is one of your problems. This problem can be moved toward positive resolution by recognizing some of your accomplishments. When you review your life with that addicted parent, you cannot help but see that you are a survivor. If you look further, you may recall managing the family budget and raising younger siblings. These clearly are accomplishments, proving you have not only done well, but are quite capable. At this point in the medicine wheel, acknowledgment of both problems and accomplishments returns balance to life. Commitment to positive growth and change provides the path to healing.

### Step 3: Beginning Today I Will Examine The Ways In Which I Have Tried To Manipulate, Control Or Manage The Lives Of Others And Make A Commitment To Stop This Behavior

This step has a great deal of meaning for recovering addicts, adult children of alcoholics, co-dependent persons and those from dysfunctional families in general. In this

step, the person who is manipulating, controlling or attempting to manage the lives of others must realize that
he or she is bringing harm to self and others, as well as
infringing on another person's sacred existence.

This might be very difficult for adult children of alcoholics or co-dependent persons to understand. The question you might ask is, "What will happen if I just allow
that other person to go on drinking and drugging?" However, the question that really needs to be asked seriously
is, "What has my over-attention to that person's addiction
accomplished?" The point here is that a co-dependent individual or an adult child of an alcoholic must realize that
she or he cannot cure addiction in that other person. In
fact, the over-attention given to the addiction only makes
the problem worse.

When the co-dependent or ACoA makes excuses for
the chemically addicted individual, that person is given
unspoken approval and support for the continuation of
the addiction. When the co-dependent person takes over
responsibilities for the addicted partner, parent or friend,
that person does not need to face the consequences of his
or her alcohol or drug use so the addiction continues.

The addictive process can only be stopped when the
chemically dependent person is left to face the consequences of his or her alcohol/drug abuse. Likewise, a co-
dependent person or an adult child of an alcoholic will
begin recovery only after releasing her or himself from
the responsibility for the impossible task of curing the
chemically addicted person. When attempts to control addiction in another person cease, when the pleading and
manipulation have ended, when the responsibility for managing his or her life is returned to the addicted person,
then and only then can the co-dependent person or the
ACoA begin recovery.

If you are a recovering addict or actively in your addiction, you need to review the ways in which you interact
with others. Do you attempt to induce guilt in others so
they won't leave you? Do you use blackmail tactics, such

as threatening to take your own life? Do you threaten another person with physical violence just to keep him or her under your control? If so, you need to make a commitment to stop this behavior. Your own recovery cannot progress until this behavior ceases. You need to stop attempting to manage others and focus on taking responsibility for your own life, your own recovery. Others cannot be blamed for your addiction and they cannot be made responsible for your sobriety.

### Step 4: Beginning Today I Will Acknowledge That Change In My Life Must Begin With Me

This step is an action step in which you empower yourself to make positive life changes. At this point on the medicine wheel, you need to acknowledge that no one can make your life changes for you. If you are waiting for a parent to stop drinking before you go on with your life, realize that you are counting on another person's changes to free you. Instead you need to say, "Today I begin the necessary work that will free me from the addiction of my parent. I am not responsible for his or her addiction and I am not at fault for never having cured his or her disease."

If you are a person who is addicted to any chemical substance, you need to realize that change begins with you. No one else can stop your addiction. Yes, others can help you, encourage you, support you, but only you can stop your addictive process. Your statement needs to be, "I cannot wait around for the right time, the magical cure, the person who will save me from me. To save my own life I must change. I have to stop abusing drugs/alcohol and begin to put my life together again. Freedom from my addiction begins today with me."

The larger meaning of this step is that regardless of the problem in your past or present (i.e., addiction, growing up in a dysfunctional family, being in a relationship with an addicted person or having no sense of meaning or direction in life) changes in your life begin with you. Walk

through the medicine wheel. Discover your personal path
to recovery. Freedom from addiction or the pain of a dysfunctional childhood can be yours. Walk the medicine
wheel way. My love goes with you.

# 3

# Positive
# Transcendence

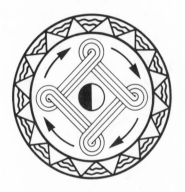

*"Awareness is like a never-ending journey into a
new land. Every time you reach the top of the mountain, you discover whole new valleys and rivers and
hills that are waiting to be explored."*

Eva Kennedy/Onieda/Michigan, 1984.

*Positive transcendence* means being transformed as a person. It means growing beyond addiction, fear, shame, guilt and anger.

*Positive transcendence* means restructuring your approach to life in a way that will help you feel powerful, capable and able to move through recovery to spiritual, physical, emotional and psychological growth. What this process will require of you is a commitment to go beyond recognition of your addiction, co-dependency or dysfunctional childhood to a real desire for inner peace, self-affirmation and a sense of wholeness.

## Balance

The cornerstone of positive transcendence is balance. Balance is part of the Recovery Medicine Wheel at many points and in many ways. There is a good reason for this.

Recovering people need to work hard at bringing balance into their lives. This balance is often lacking in persons, relationships or family systems affected by drugs or alcohol. Simply removing chemical substances from your life does not mean you have returned to a more balanced existence. Reading literature on characteristics of ACoAs may make you knowledgeable about why you act the way you do, but if this same knowledge is not used to bring about positive changes, your life remains unbalanced.

### Why Is It So Important To Achieve Balance?

Without balance, we are easily affected by life stresses in ways that can lead to relapse. For co-dependent people and adult children of alcoholics, relapse might mean a return to self-destructive behavioral patterns such as involvement in intimate relationships with emotionally abusive people. ACoA or co-dependent relapse also could bring a return to self-hatred, feelings of failure, attempts to be a "fixer" of other people's lives, resumption of compulsive work patterns or denial of feelings.

For chemically dependent people, relapse may begin with feelings of self-hatred but is soon dealt with in the old familiar way . . . a return to substance abuse. Chemically dependent people also deny feelings of depression, fear, loneliness and anger, but they deny it through the use of chemical substances. Pain is unbearable and medication of pain is seen as the only reasonable alternative.

Your view of life becomes narrow when the balance is lost. When the view of life becomes narrow, growth and learning cease. When growth and learning cease, stagnation occurs. Stagnation is followed by boredom, boredom by depression, depression by self-hatred and anger, and self-hatred and anger by relapse. Therefore, the maintenance of balance is most important. For without balance, the likelihood of relapse is high.

### But What About Balance? How Is It Achieved And Maintained?

The methods of maintaining balance in life are numerous. If you follow the steps of the Recovery Medicine Wheel, you will have a basic guideline for gaining an understanding of the path to balance. But before we speak of applying the Recovery Medicine Wheel for balance, let us examine unbalanced approaches to recovery.

A recovering ACoA once said to me, "My mom doesn't drink anymore but she's still addictive as hell." When I asked him to describe what he meant, he said, "At her house, you can have any type of breakfast cereal you want as long as it is Raisin Bran, Raisin Bran or Raisin Bran." He told me how his mother had closed off all contacts with former friends and stopped engaging in the activities she used to enjoy. He said he was afraid she would relapse and he would be dragged into her addiction again as a caretaker.

Clearly, both persons in this scenario were in need of balance. Although his mom's dietary habits were portrayed by the young man in a rather comical way, he was still trying to make a serious point. He was saying that although his mother was no longer drinking alcohol, she was still living in an addictive fashion in other areas of her life.

What is the point here? First, Mom needs to recognize
the danger in continuing with addictive life patterns. Sec-
ondly, son is in need of refocusing his approach to his
mother's struggles with recovery. By his own admission,
this man was on his way to relapse as a caretaker.

At this point you are likely saying, "Fine, I can see the
relapse coming. I can see the need for balance. But what
should these people do?" For starters, the son needs to
remember that he is not responsible for his mother's addiction and he cannot cure her, force her to recover against
her will or make her acquire balance in her life. In addition,
he should not deny his sadness, anger, fear or disappointment at seeing his mother set herself up for relapse. What
he can do is calmly discuss with his mother the danger
signals he sees. He also must be prepared to have his mother retaliate with anger, denial and/or a combination of pla-
cation (you're worried about nothing) or rationalization (Raisin Bran is the only thing that tastes good to me).

If this young man would return to the medicine wheel
and read it carefully, he would see that releasing himself
from responsibility for his mother's addiction is one of the
changes he must make in his life if he truly seeks a balanced existence.

On the other hand, Mom needs to recognize that her
sobriety and recovery are in trouble. Mom needs to be
aware that by limiting her diet, she is creating an unbalanced condition in her body. Without certain nutrients in
her system, she could begin to feel lethargic, even depressed. This down feeling could in turn lead to relapse
(Mueller and Ketcham, 1987).

Another way to understand the negative effects of un-
balanced living is communicated through the story of
Peach Tree. I am not sure where the story originated, but
I will tell it to you as it was told to me.

### The Story Of Peach Tree

There existed at one time, long ago, a big beautiful peach
tree. This peach tree lived in a wide grassy canyon near a deep
clear river.

One day a young boy discovered Peach Tree and picked and ate one of the peaches. The young boy exclaimed out loud, "What a delicious peach and what a beautiful tree!" Soon everyone in the village was making trips to pick peaches. Peach Tree was very happy. All summer she gave her peaches away to the people. When fall arrived, however, all the peaches were gone. The people of the village stopped coming to see Peach Tree and this made Peach Tree very sad.

All summer, she had heard people talk beneath her, picking and eating her peaches and saying how much they loved her, but now no one came around. The people were busy with other things. They were hunting elk, gathering wood and drying squash for the winter ahead.

All fall and winter Peach Tree stood alone with no more than an occasional visitor. Finally spring arrived and Peach Tree burst into beautiful dark pink blossoms. Her perfume filled the air and young girls from the village came to smell her flowers and share secrets beneath her shady branches. It was then that Peach Tree decided she would not stop giving away, not even when fall and winter arrived.

As summer came and went, Peach Tree kept producing peaches. She was happy to be giving away to the people. Every day, the villagers would visit her and go home with many peaches. As Peach Tree wanted all the people to love her and be near her, she spent all her time making peaches. She did nothing but make peaches. Peach Tree never wanted the people to leave her alone again, so she worked night and day to make and give away as many peaches as she possibly could.

One day in late summer, River said, "Peach Tree, you must take water or you will die."

Peach Tree replied, "I need no water. I am fine. If I stop to take water, I will have to quit making and giving away peaches. If I do that, the people will leave. Maybe later I will take water."

After River spoke, Mother Earth talked to Peach Tree. "Peach Tree, you have taken no food from the soil. If you take no food, you will die."

Again Peach Tree replied, "I am fine. I am too busy making peaches to stop and take food from the soil. If I do that, I will have to stop making peaches and if that happens, the people will leave."

Peach Tree went on through the fall making peaches. Every day, people would visit her and they would be amazed at all the peaches she was producing.

As winter approached, Wind came to speak to Peach Tree. "Peach Tree, you need to sleep now. If you try to stay awake all winter, you will freeze to death. Only if you sleep like the river, frogs and bears will you make it through the cold season. Look, you have not even made new buds for the spring."

Peach Tree replied, "I am fine. I have to make peaches. If I don't make peaches, the people will leave me alone again. I have to keep giving away."

Finally Winterman came to the canyon. The air became very cold. Soon all the peaches froze and fell to the ground. Peach Tree's leaves turned brown and dropped. When the people from the village saw what had happened, they stopped visiting the tree. Soon the dead peaches turned brown and even the birds did not come. Now Peach Tree was all alone. She had many dead and frost-blistered branches. Winter was well underway and Peach Tree was freezing to death.

One day in early spring, a small bird landed on Peach Tree. The bird could hear Peach Tree singing her death song. Immediately the bird flew away to the village. The bird told the people that Peach Tree was singing her death song.

Since the people loved Peach Tree, they came out once more to the river where she lived. The people made a circle around Peach Tree and began to sing a song. As they sang the healing song, Peach Tree could feel life flowing back into her branches. Soon all the branches had tight little buds on them. Peach Tree could feel the water entering into her roots. She could feel the food pouring into her from Mother Earth. It was then that Peach Tree understood that the people loved her, not just when she was giving away peaches, but also when she was blooming or sleeping or turning red in the fall.

With the love of the people, Peach Tree had returned from sickness to health. Through the love of River, Mother Earth, Wind and the people, Peach Tree learned that she must allow herself to take water, food and rest. She discovered that only through taking good care of herself would she be able to give away to others.

The bottom line is to maintain balance in all areas of life. This balance will create fertile ground for growth in a positive direction.

## Is Your Life Out Of Balance?

If you are confused about balance, return to the Recovery Medicine Wheel. Read the steps. Discuss the steps with others, and watch for these key warning signs that indicate your life is out of balance.

1. Has your diet become very limited for reasons other than shortage of food or money to purchase food?
2. Are you eating more sugar?
3. Has your coffee-drinking or cigarette-smoking increased?
4. Are you overworking (arriving at work early, staying late, skipping lunch or dinner)?
5. Have you placed exercise or relaxation last on your list of priorities?
6. Have you begun to assume more responsibilities at work or at home because you feel no one else will do them or they won't do them correctly?
7. Has your thinking become very negative regarding yourself and life in general?
8. Do you feel defeated, tired, uncreative, incompetent, etc.?
9. Have you given up on your physical and mental health resolutions one by one?
10. Do you feel the need to make sweeping, total, drastic life changes immediately? For example, do you think you should quit your job, pack your bags, load up the car and move across the country tomorrow?
11. Do you see learning, growing and working at maintaining balance in your life as too hard and not worth the trouble?
12. Do you see yourself looking for the quick fix, the short-cut to solving the problem or attaining your goals?
13. Are you thinking you should give up on trying to live a healthy positive life because you feel, "It was a stupid idea to believe I could change or be happy anyway"?
14. Do you find yourself engaging in obsessive thinking (primarily negative) that leaves you feeling out of control or scared? (For example, are you constantly afraid that you might return to drinking or drugging? Are you perhaps concerned with finding a safe place, getting control of yourself and making the right life choices now? Do you find yourself feeling

fearful, wanting to run and not being able to identify where these frightening feelings are coming from? Most importantly, are these thoughts going through your mind day and night with very little relief? If so, you are caught in obsessive thinking.)

If you see these signs in yourself, you are clearly out of balance. To restore balance and proper perspective to your existence, look again to the Recovery Medicine Wheel. Try to understand the many ways in which the wheel speaks of balance. Follow this with making decisions about changes that will lead you back to balance.

If you are overworking, explore methods of lightening your work load. If you find yourself making hasty or poorly planned life choices, slow down and look at the ramifications of your decisions. Gain information, understand clearly what your life choices will involve, what at least some of the consequences will be. Be extremely wary of any life directional choice . . . a career move, a geographic move or involvement in a relationship with another person . . . in which you are unable to see the bad with the good.

Remember, if something looks and sounds too good to be true, it probably is. This does not mean that a situational or relationship choice may not be a move in a more positive direction; it simply means that no relationship or situation is perfect. It may be better . . . but it won't be perfect. This needs to be made clear in your own mind. For if you embark upon any major life change expecting everything to be just fine, you are setting yourself up for disappointment, disillusionment and disaster. On the other hand, if you understand that change brings with it the need to adjust to new circumstances, your expectations are more realistic and, therefore, more balanced.

When you apply the Recovery Medicine Wheel to your life in search of balance, start by remembering that it is a tool with which you can center yourself. The Recovery Medicine Wheel will not bring you back to balance if you act as a passive participant just along for the ride. It can serve only as guide. *You* must walk through the steps of the wheel, listen to the words and choose your direction. *You* must take an active part in seeking to regain balance in your life.

## How To Find Balance

To begin this process, read each step of the wheel carefully. Often one or more of the steps will seem to leap out at you, to speak directly to you, to address the feeling you are having at this moment.

Let us assume, for example, that you have read through the 14 warning signs mentioned earlier and find that you feel the need to make drastic life changes immediately. In this case, a number of steps in the Recovery Medicine Wheel will apply to your current situation. First, the fourth step in the North will likely strike you as very relevant to your present unbalanced state. That step reads: *"Beginning today I will come to an understanding that change is a process (I can't expect miracles overnight)."*

Reading this step, thinking about it and perhaps discussing it with others, can help you to regain balance and centeredness because it stresses the word *process*. Changing your life for the better is a process. If you want to be better educated, you must go through the process of attending class, taking tests, writing papers, reading books. If you plan to improve your health, you will need to change eating habits, develop exercise and relaxation routines and begin the process of returning your body to a state of well-being. No substantive life change will be achieved instantly. To know, understand and accept meaningful change is a process achieved over time.

The process of regaining balance in your life involves looking at many different areas of your existence. You need to look at what you are saying to and about yourself, the way you are behaving in your interaction with others and the way you are thinking.

## 6 Helpful Steps To Bring Back Balance

1. Recognition of your current unbalanced state is the first and most important step. Read the 14 warning signs mentioned earlier.
2. Seek out people (your recovery group) or a person (a therapist or friend) who can help you see where and how you are being overly negative in assessing yourself.
3. Make and carrying out plans to nurture your own spirit, be it through meditation, praying, chanting or simply being alone in a place where you have traditionally felt happy or content. The place you choose to be alone can be by a lake, an ocean, out in the desert, near a stream in the mountains, in the forest, beside a river or even in your own garden. The act of taking time to be alone with the earth and your own thoughts in a healing place will allow you to let go of some of the negativity that has you out of balance.
4. Plan healthy, constructive and enjoyable activities for yourself. Some examples of healthy, constructive activities are going to a good movie, attending a stage play, cooking a gourmet meal, horseback riding, swimming, dancing, skiing, fishing, painting or even something as simple as chopping wood. The important thing to remember is that the activity be healthy, constructive and enjoyable.
5. To balance yourself in the Recovery Medicine Wheel way, read each step carefully. Think about how each step applies to your life and your current situation. Discuss the Recovery Medicine Wheel with supportive people to gain a greater understanding of the steps and in bringing yourself back into a state of balance. Work the steps of the Recovery Medicine Wheel on a regular basis (usually daily).
6. Stick with your commitments made as a result of going through this rebalancing process. Remember that regaining balance will not happen instantly. As the Recovery Medicine Wheel states, *"Change is a*

*process."* After all, you didn't get out of balance instantly. You will not regain balance instantly either.

The process of recovery will have its ups and downs. Be prepared for some disappointments and periods of time when progress seems slow or nonexistent. Setbacks and slowdowns are all part of the unavoidable pitfalls encountered in recovery.

A good example of what I am talking about is the case of a woman we will call Susan. When talking about her recovery, Susan often compares her early stages of recovery to her present state of living.

"At first, balanced living was so difficult," she said. "It felt good, but foreign, real foreign. For so many years I had been isolating myself. I would get lonely and afraid and knew the booze would help me escape. But finally the booze didn't work anymore. Balanced living, the way of Mother Earth, was my only choice, that is, my only choice besides death or another addiction.

"Every day I would look at the Recovery Medicine Wheel, read the steps and it would feel good for a while, but then the old feelings and fears would come back. So back to the wheel I would go. I must have read that wheel ten times a day when I started. I even centered my individual counseling sessions on the steps of the Recovery Medicine Wheel. Those first few months were rough. I even relapsed twice, but each time I got up, brushed myself off and started again.

"After about four months of good, solid sobriety, I felt the balance coming into my life. The way of the Recovery Medicine Wheel became easier. My life was starting to move with rhythm. I became more aware of the world around me and noticed that I reached out more to other people.

"That was almost two years ago. Now when I have problems, I look for lots of different ways to solve the problem. I get together with my support group. I go out

to my spot near the river to meditate. I exercise, read my
Recovery Medicine Wheel and do lots of things.

"You see, I don't just do one thing to solve a problem, I do
many different things; I balance it all out. If one way doesn't
work, I look for another. But what is more important than
that is my balance in all areas of life. I take time to take care
of my spirit, my mind and my body. When I am getting
negative, I use positive self-statements. When I feel restless,
I get in touch with my spiritual self. I also make sure I take
care of my body. I have learned to love myself and I think
this all comes from the balanced way of living.

"Balance has become natural. It's kind of funny, but
now that old drunk, frightened me is foreign. I have really
changed and, believe me, if I can change from the old me
to the way I am now, I know other people can do it too.
Balance . . . that's the key . . . balance."

Just like a baby who is learning to walk, you, too, will
wobble or stumble out of balance from time to time. But
just as babies grow more able to walk unencumbered,
you, too, will grow in your ability to achieve and maintain
balance. As balance becomes your way of living, your recovery will feel more natural. So work toward balance
and have trust. Change is possible and, as Susan said,
"Balance . . . that's the key . . . balance."

## Harmony (Seeking Inner Peace)

Harmony is something many people speak of but few
understand. You may have heard of harmony referred to
in the context of the relationship between humans and
their environment. Perhaps you have heard mental health
professionals speak of harmonious relations between
spouses or members of a family.

When you hear the word *harmony*, you may even think
of people singing. Whatever the case, harmony is a word
you are familiar with, but the concept may remain difficult
to grasp. Like happiness, harmony is not something that
can be sought or arrived at directly. Harmony is a by-
product of spiritual, physical, emotional and psychological

well-being. Harmony is a state of inner peace and contentment that results from healthy balance in all areas of living.

Harmony within the spirit and body of any recovering person is an essential element in the overall process of healthy living. Harmony gives the recovering person a sense of inner peace. You are now free to use your energies to be creative. As a result of this rediscovered energy, solving the problems of everyday living becomes easier. This is not because your problems have been made more manageable, but because you now have an increased ability to think of creative solutions.

Look at it this way. If you plan to build a house and you have only a hammer, the job will be difficult. On the other hand, if you have an entire box of tools, a truck and a cement mixer the job will be much easier. The house has not changed at all. The blueprints are the same. The materials that need to be pieced together are identical. What has changed, however, is your ability to put the house together properly. Achieving a state of harmony, of inner peace, is like increasing the number of tools available to you.

### How Is Harmony Achieved?

How can you get this sense of inner peace? Remember, harmony, like happiness, cannot be pursued directly. It is a by-product of healthy, balanced, integrated living.

As you become more able to maintain balance, you will experience a calmness that feels very much like a strong smooth river flowing inside you. This river of energy and strength is the feeling of harmony. When harmony is present, a sensation of almost electrifying, positive, creative energy will be felt. This sensation will not and does not have the shallow, superficial satisfaction of alcohol, drugs, compulsively eaten food or dependent relationships. It is something deeper. It is a whole, pure, complete sensation. The feeling of living in harmony is not a sudden rush of euphoria that soon fades. It is strong and sustained, and leaves you feeling whole in a way that no form of instant gratification can. A drug lets you crash. A state of harmony sustains you.

There are certain things you can do that will make experiencing harmony more likely. First, the continuation of addictions and addictive life patterns must be recognized and stopped. If you are addicted to any chemical substance, that substance must be removed from your life before a state of harmony can come about. However, other more subtle or socially acceptable forms of addictive living must change as well.

For example, a person who devotes all of his or her time to work may be seen by peers and society as a successful person, an achiever. Many people may comment that such a person is a workaholic, but few will admit that this same person has a real addiction. After all, she or he is successful, drives a nice car, wears nice clothes, etc. She or he doesn't fit at all with our society's stereotyped view of an addicted person. We see the workaholic as doing okay. But is she or he? The workaholic may suffer from high blood pressure, heart disease, ulcers and a myriad of other physical and mental problems.

Likewise, a woman who is the complete self-sacrificing caregiver of her family and/or spouse is often seen by society as a totally loving and caring person, to some a saint. Yet this same person may have feelings of depression, loneliness and fear. She often has no self-defined image, no core identity outside of that associated with her role as a spouse, mother, aunt or caregiver.

People such as those described above are not experiencing a state of harmonious living but they are living within accepted norms. So why should they change?

They should change for themselves. Does this sound selfish to you? It isn't. Think of some of the happiest, most self-assured people you have met. These are the people who have taken time to nurture their own spirits, to balance all areas of their lives. These are the ones who seem to have boundless energy and incredible inner strength. That is because they are living in harmony.

Think for a moment what being around such people does for you. It gives you a sense of being at ease. Such people will draw others to them. Well-balanced individuals living in a state of harmony are able to share themselves freely. The net result of all of this is that many others will benefit in a positive way from contact with those who are in harmony with themselves and their world.

If you believe people won't like you because you take time to care for yourself, think of what you have just read. Yes, some might not be pleased with your growth and change, but these are people who want you to stay in your caretaking, dependent or overachieving role because it serves some particular purpose for them. In the long run, those relationships or lifestyles that you develop out of love (for yourself as well as others) will be far more satisfying than those born of fear, loneliness and dependency.

Dave had spent many years as the caretaker of his family. In describing his situation, Dave told me, "I was trying to do everything. I wanted the family to have some kind of order, so I spent all my time trying to make things right.

"We lived in the country and didn't have a lot of money, so there was always work to do just to keep things going. I had wood to chop, meals to cook, clothes to wash and the animals to take care of. I was always busy, always tired and always worried."

In describing his family, Dave also talked about his parents and the way both of them had turned over the responsibility of running the family to him. Dave always tried to look his best and present the best image of his family to the community. Dave played this caretaker role for most of his teenage and early adult years. It wasn't until age 26 that he finally sought some help.

After years of dealing with his alcoholic parents, Dave sank into a deep depression. At one point, he himself had started to drink and even thought of committing suicide. He recalls a poem that he shared with his therapist after his third session. The poem reads as follows:

## *Death Of A Dream*

*I'm just a stone on a stormy strand and waves*
*have ground me into sand.*
*The icy seas have crystal knives, they cut my*
*flesh and drain my life.*
*They melt away with breaking dawn. The*
*wounds remain, the knives are gone.*
*Oh, let me sleep an endless night by flickering*
*tongues of firelight.*
*My soul no longer waits for dawn.*
*The eagle is dead.*
*My dream is gone.*
*I feel a hundred years of age. A grass fire*
*burned has lost its rage.*
*A blackened prairie waits for rain to stop the*
*smoke, and ease the pain.*

Clearly the years Dave spent trying to "fix" his family had taken their toll. Dave became depressed, suicidal and was having his own problems with alcohol. With the help of his therapist and the discovery of the Recovery Medicine Wheel, he started to feel better emotionally. He realized the need to take care of himself. He had to give up his belief that he could "cure" his parents and make everything right in the family.

He had to restore balance to his life. He had to do less for others and more for himself. Why? Because his own life was being drained.

Look at his poem again. Dave's spirit was depleted. He never took time to fill himself back up again. He left himself empty and lost. As a caretaker and a martyr, Dave may have looked noble and caring to others, but he was out of balance and he was destroying his most precious gift . . . his spirit.

If you desire a state of harmony or inner peace, pay close attention to balance in all areas of living. Walk the steps of the Recovery Medicine Wheel. Think of what each step means to you and how the wheel can be applied in your life. Recognize that both harmony and balance are spoken of in many ways and at many points on the Recovery Medicine Wheel. It is critically important that you address your needs in all areas of living: physical, emotional, psychological and spiritual.

## Maintaining Balance

Think of driving a car. You can't just start your automobile, point it in the direction you want to go and take off. Rather, you need to make constant small adjustments with the steering wheel, give it more gas when you go up a hill, brake when you reach a stop sign and so forth. When you begin to see balancing your life as a process of adjustments (some minor, some major), you will be better able to move and grow in a positive direction.

An improved self-concept will allow you to feel more competent and capable. Your positivity will allow you to release yourself from burdensome fear, anger, loneliness and anxiety. As time passes and as you become better able to adjust to life circumstances by responding to change with healthy adaptations, you will begin to experience that feeling of self-assuredness, of calmness.

With the Recovery Medicine Wheel as a guide, these healthy adaptations to living will be more easily recognized and put into operation. Your recovery group, your therapist or trusted other and your own insight will help you unravel the meaning of each step of the Recovery Medicine Wheel.

As you walk the Recovery Medicine Wheel path, you will learn to understand yourself better. You will begin to see new ways of working through problems. You will find that the old path, the way of addiction, is not the only choice you have. You no longer will be trapped by the need to deny feelings, rationalize behavior and return to substance abuse.

Just as the sun brings new light to the earth each morning, working the steps of the Recovery Medicine Wheel will help you shed light on new ideas. It will illuminate the path to self-discovery and personal growth that you may have forgotten, or perhaps have never known. When this occurs, inner peace will be experienced; harmony will be a reality.

One caution: Do not become discouraged if harmony seems fleeting, especially at first. Just work at balancing your life. In time, balancing will become easier and harmony less fleeting. But remember, change is a process; don't expect miracles overnight. Work steadily at developing a healthy lifestyle for yourself. Living in harmony is something you can experience. It is a way of existing that is within your grasp through balanced living. Use the steps of the Recovery Medicine Wheel to find understanding, to gain knowledge of yourself and the world around you. *Find yourself, find your path, seek the truth of your existence and inner peace will come to you.*

## Centeredness

Having centeredness in life means discovering, or perhaps rediscovering, your core self. To be centered is to have a deep spiritual understanding of your place in the world, your connection to all of creation. This does not mean finding out who you are in terms of other people. Rather, having centeredness means discovering who you are to yourself.

As an old Ojibwa Indian man from Canada once told me, "I may wear these plastic moccasins, and I would probably tip over into the water if I tried to cross the St. Mary's River in a canoe, but I know what is in my heart." At that point he held up a cane. On the end of the cane was tied an eagle feather. The old gentleman raised his hand up under the feather, allowing it to rest softly in his palm. He continued:

> You see, in my heart I know I am part of this beautiful creation. Many people wear the clothes and sing the songs. They say this makes them real Indians. But what does that mean? Clothes and songs are just that: clothes and songs. If you do not feel the connection to your creation, to this beautiful Mother Earth, doing and saying all the right things will mean nothing. It is what you feel in your heart that matters. Everything else is like actors in a play.

It might sound nice, it might look nice, but it isn't real.

Although this meeting occurred years ago, the words of that elder have stayed with me ever since. His message of my need to understand my spiritual self, my connection to all of creation, has helped me define who I am.

"But," you might ask, "how did you do that; how did you come to know your connection to all of creation and how can I do the same? What path must I follow to find my spirituality, my core, my self?"

First, finding your true self calls for a great deal of work. It requires meditation, questioning your own beliefs and seeking knowledge. Finding your true self means going beyond the labels you have had placed upon you by yourself or society. Finding what is in your heart, what exists beyond the clothes and songs, takes a desire to seek truth.

For example, if you attend church or engage in ceremonies simply because others will see you and say you are a good person, are you really doing what is in your heart? Are you following your own spiritual path, or are you just going through the motions that are expected of you by family, friends or society?

On the other hand, if you offer tobacco leaves to the river because you are thankful to share in the moment, even if no one else is around, then you are following your heart. Likewise, if you burst into song, tears or dance at the sight of a beautiful sunset, you are experiencing the truth of your spirituality. Perhaps a story about the "trickster" would help clarify this discussion of spirituality.

## The Trickster

Among many tribes of Native American people, traditional stories include the teachings of a trickster. The trickster is often a spirit who is represented in the form of an animal. In certain tribes, the trickster is a coyote, in others a rabbit and in still others, the trickster is a raven. In this particular story (from the Ottawa tribe), the trickster is Waboozoo (Rabbit). His antics are meant to entertain the listener while teaching a lesson.

## Waboozoo And The Three Blind Men

Waboozoo (Rabbit) decided one day that he would play a trick on the three old blind men who lived near the river. The three men had a rope that ran from their house to the river. Each day one of the blind men would follow the rope to the river, fill a bucket with water and return to the house. They had lived this way for many years and had become accustomed to living in their little cabin by the river.

One day Waboozoo said to himself, "I want to stir things up for those complacent old men." So he went down to the river and untied the rope, took the end of the rope and tied it to a jack pine tree at the edge of a sand pit.

The next morning one of the old blind men followed the rope to the river but, because of Waboozoo's trick, the rope led the old man to the sand pit instead. When the old blind man dipped his bucket into what he thought was the river, he came up with a bucket full of sand.

"Wish-ta!" said the old man. "The river has dried up!" At that point, the old man dropped the bucket and ran back along the rope to the cabin.

Waboozoo laughed and laughed. He could hear the old men yelling, "What will we do?" While the old blind men yelled at each other, Waboozoo took the rope and tied it back by the river. Just when he was done, Waboozoo heard one of the old men say, "You are just lazy. You didn't even go to the river. I will go get us water." When the second old man got to the end of the rope, there was the river. Now he was sure the other old fellow was lying. When the second old man got back to the cabin, a real shouting match started. The old men argued all morning and Waboozoo rolled on the forest floor laughing and holding his belly.

By the time night arrived, the old men had stopped arguing. However, no one was talking. The first old man and the second old man were angry at one another. The third old blind man didn't talk for fear of starting another fight. Finally, the three exhausted old men went to sleep by the crackling fire in the fireplace.

Before sunrise the next day, Waboozoo again went down to the end of the rope by the river. He untied the rope and took the loose end back to the sand pit. Again, he tied the rope to the jack pine tree. There Waboozoo waited.

When the old blind men heard the singing of many birds, they knew it was daytime. Now since the old men took turns, this was the second old man's day to get the water. He grabbed his bucket and grumbled something to the first old man but before he got an answer, he was out of the door. Still grumbling, when he got to the end of the rope, the second old man dropped his bucket down into what he thought was the river, but to his surprise, all he heard was a "clang" when the bucket hit the sand.

"Wish-ta!" yelled the old man, "The river is dry!"

By now Waboozoo was laughing so hard that tears were rolling down his cheeks. He could hear all the old men yelling and throwing things around the house. The third old man said, "You are both lazy. I'll go get the water." Again Waboozoo stopped laughing long enough to take the rope back down to the river. When the third old man got to the end of the rope, there was the river.

This time, the old man getting the water was so angry he started yelling right there at the river. He yelled and yelled. He was so loud that the other two blind men heard him back at the cabin. Because they thought something might be wrong, they followed the rope to the river. When they got there, a fight started. "I'm sick of you two. You are both lazy!" "What do you mean, lazy?" said the other two. On and on went the fight.

Suddenly one of the old blind men grabbed the other two by the arms and shouted, "Listen!" Off in the forest they could hear Waboozoo laughing.

One of the men called out to Waboozoo, "What are you laughing at?" "I am laughing at you," said Waboozoo. "You all followed the rope and nobody checked to make sure the rope was going the right way. You old blind men were so sure you were on your way to the river so that when I moved the rope around, you got mad at each other. Nobody stopped to think they were being tricked. You old men have sure given me some fun. I'll be on my way now. So long!"

And off he went, laughing as he hopped away through the trees.

What this story tells us is that following a path without question is not a good idea. In the story the old blind men represented tradition. The fact that they were blind meant that some traditions are never questioned, just accepted. The rope represented empty rituals—rituals that are followed or performed in a mechanical way. When trickster rabbit came into the picture, he was meant to trick the old blind men into learning. By moving the rope, Waboozoo was showing that traditions without meaning will cause people to argue over who is right, who follows the right way.

When Waboozoo finally revealed himself, he represented illumination, the coming of knowledge to all people
who become lost or confused by following traditions
blindly. By getting the old men to argue, Waboozoo also
showed us how people often believe their own experience
of life is the only real or valid experience.

The story of Waboozoo and the three old blind men
shows us the importance of having ritual, belief and cer-
emony that have meaning in our lives. The story also
teaches us to listen to one another. It teaches us to see
that our own truth is often not the only truth. It teaches
us to question, to search for truth and to seek illumination. With this illumination we will be able to see the
proper path to the life-giving spiritual river that flows
within each of us.

There is no specific formula, no one way to follow that
will lead to self-discovery. In fact, even the Recovery Medicine Wheel is only a guide. It can inspire you, direct you,
help you focus on a thought, but it cannot lead you because
each of us, being sacred and unique, must find a spiritual
path that is our own. We cannot depend on others to give
us the directions to the discovery of our inner selves.

The only thing that can be said here is that you will
know the path you follow is right when your connection
to creation has the quality of being energizing and uplifting. *When the "earth song," that spiritual energy that emanates
from the mother of us all, can be felt vibrating inside of you, you
will know your core, your spiritual self; you will have centeredness.*

## Freedom

Like all medicine wheels, the Recovery Medicine Wheel
is a mirror for each person. For example, if you look at the
first step in the West (the realm of introspective thought)
you will read: "Beginning today I will speak honestly with
myself." Different people will react in very different ways
to this step. Some may say, "I don't know how or where to
start." Others may say, "I am afraid to speak honestly
with myself." Some might even feel they are not ready for

or capable of self-honesty at this time. Whatever the case may be, your reaction to each step of the Recovery Medicine Wheel will be a clue for you, a mirror.

It is that mirroring that will help you find the proper path to recovery. As you explore yourself through the Recovery Medicine Wheel, your reflections will help you grow and change, to heal, to recover, to continually gain freedom from the behaviors that hold you back in life.

Many of us have traditionally thought of freedom in terms of physical/geographical movement or financial security. These are only facets of overall or complete freedom. Some people move about, travel great distances, have glamorous professions or a great deal of financial wealth. Nevertheless, many of these same people are not free. They often suffer from fear, anxiety, loneliness or self-hatred.

Why is this so? It is so because these people do not have emotional, psychological or spiritual freedom to go along with their physical good fortune. To be free you need to explore and understand your past.

- Are you still consumed by anger and resentment over what may have happened to you as a child of an alcoholic or drug-addicted parent?
- Do you still hate yourself, or feel used or like a fool for being or having been in a co-dependent role in a relationship with another person?
- Are you often overcome with guilt for the suffering you have caused your loved ones during the active phase of your addiction?

Well, as long as these feelings, ways of thinking and self-perceptions exist, you cannot be free. It will always feel as though you are tied down or held back from becoming the person you would like to be. What needs to be done here is to allow yourself to see these ways of thinking and the behaviors that go with them as mirrors.

In the mirror of guilt, for example, you can see yourself clearly. You can see yourself as a person who is ashamed, as a person who feels of little or no worth. To see yourself in the mirror of guilt is to see a person in emotional pain. If you will see this pain for what it is, understand why the guilt is there and make the necessary changes in your life, you will begin the process of freeing yourself.

For example, let us say that you have a lot of unresolved guilt over the treatment of your children during the active phase of your addiction. Why are you feeling guilty? Perhaps you inflicted a great deal of emotional pain on your family while you were drugging or drinking and you now fear that serious emotional damage has been done. What can you do? You can speak openly with your children about your addiction. You can let them know that you are sorry. You also can help your children find their own paths to recovery through therapy, support groups and reading.

When this has been done, you will need to say to yourself, "I have made amends to my children. I have directed them to people and places that will help them recover and now I must get on with my own recovery."

Remember, you can only assist your loved ones in recovery by directing them to those resources that will help (therapists, recovery groups, books). You cannot "cure" them. Just as you are responsible for your own recovery, so are they for theirs. *You can help them find the path to recovery, but you cannot walk it for them.*

## Letting Go

What all this means is that you need to learn how to let go of your emotional pain. For as long as you hold onto your pain, you cannot continue growing and changing as a person. Emotional pain must be recognized, understood, worked through and released.

Think of what would happen to an aspen tree if it never lost its leaves in the fall. Soon the tree would become crowded with dead leaves. New leaves would not be able to grow because all the space would be taken up by the dead leaves the tree would not release. Eventually, the tree would die. It is the same with your spirit. If you hold onto old pain and problems, if you never let go of your anger and resentment, no new growth will occur and your spirit eventually will stagnate and die. So the key here is to process your pain, anger, resentment, guilt or whatever and then let it go.

For example, if you are an ACoA who still feels fearful when it comes to attempting new or different ways of living, you need to acknowledge that fear, work through it and let your fear go.

Remember, it is okay if you try something new and fall flat on your face; you are allowed to make mistakes. Have you ever seen a baby who gives up trying to walk because she fell down once? Of course not; she tries again and again, each time learning from her mistakes and modifying her approach. So if you try something new, say a career change, and it doesn't work out, chalk it up to experience. At least now you know what you don't like and this will make it a little easier next time you venture forth to try something new.

Most recovering people have a tendency to give up on new approaches to life very quickly. As a result, they often retreat to what is safe, what is known. However, when they retreat rapidly from fear in fear, it isn't long before they become angry with themselves, feel like failures and begin that downward negative spiral that leads to self-hatred, boredom or perhaps, in the case of recovering addicts, a return to chemical substance abuse.

## What Is The Freedom You, As A Recovering Person, Need To Seek?

Stated simply, you need to find healthy and constructive ways of releasing yourself from fear, anger, self-hatred, guilt, shame or whatever is keeping you from becoming a person with a positive sense of self, a person with a sense of wholeness and inner peace. However, to achieve personal freedom from the emotional backlog you carry with you from day to day, certain steps must be taken. In processing and releasing your emotions, you need to learn:

1. How to recognize what is going on inside you.
2. How to experience or feel your emotions.
3. How to let those pent-up emotions go.

To assist you in going through this process, consider the suggestions listed below:

### 1. *Read each step of the Recovery Medicine Wheel carefully and note your reactions.*

Remember that your responses to the steps are clues to what is going on inside of you. Let your reactions to the Recovery Medicine Wheel become mirrors, mirrors within which you can see yourself clearly. When you can do this and be honest with yourself about what you see, you will be taking the first step toward personal freedom.

### 2. *Give yourself permission to feel.*

Most recovering people have learned only too well how to shut off and deny their own feelings. Whether the desire is to cry, yell or laugh joyfully, you need to allow a means of expression for these feelings that come from the very core of your being. If you are sad, angry, happy or content, let yourself experience that emotion. Don't deny your feelings by denying yourself the opportunity of experiencing them. If you want to laugh, laugh from your core. If tears begin to surface, don't throw up that familiar dam. Instead, let them flow naturally. Tell yourself that all your emotions are valid, from laughter and caring to anger and sadness. Remember, it is in feeling that we know we are human, we know we are alive.

### 3. *Release your emotions.*

To be free of the anxiety, fear, depression or whatever might cripple you emotionally, you must learn how to release what is pent up inside of you. To release anger (in ways that will not inflict physical or emotional pain) you can walk, jog or run until you are exhausted. You also can find an open field with no one around and yell out loud.

You even can learn to use relaxation and meditation to release anger. For anxiety and fear, you can close your eyes and visualize yourself releasing those emotions to the wind or the river. You even can imagine your spirit being washed clean by the waves of a lake or ocean.

There are many ways, times and places that will allow you to release your emotions, and release is the key to freedom from that which limits you or holds you back. Remember that as long as you hold your feelings in, they will be as dead leaves are to the aspen tree. They will continue to grow thicker and heavier until no room exists for anything new. However, when you learn to let go, you will know renewal; you will experience spiritual, psychological, emotional and physical revitalization. *When you are able to recognize, feel and release what is within you, you will understand freedom.*

## Positive Transcendence

With balance, harmony, centeredness and freedom together, the means by which you can grow beyond your addiction, beyond your past, are made clearer. The four elements of positive transcendence build on the concepts of the Recovery Medicine Wheel and thereby make it better understood. Through positive transcendence the Recovery Medicine Wheel is clarified. Through the steps of the Recovery Medicine Wheel positive transcendence is actualized. Through your own awakening, recovery is realized.

# 4

# The Optimal Recovery Model

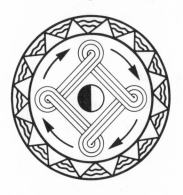

*"For me all of the pieces of my life come together when I take the teachings of the elders and I make them a real part of my existence in today's world."*

*Peggy Romero/Laguna Pueblo/New Mexico, 1988.*

The effects of addiction are serious and profound, touching not only those individuals directly involved in the disease process, but family, friends and lovers as well. The dysfunction that addiction brings to human systems leaves deep and lasting emotional scars. For this reason recovery is a difficult process, whether for ACoAs, co-dependent or chemically dependent people. Fear, insecurity, low sense of self-confidence or self-worth all combine to make "rooting out" old dysfunctional behaviors extremely problematic. Therefore, any approach to recovery must tackle the problem of dysfunctional living from a number of different angles.

The optimal recovery model presented in this chapter is an approach to recovery that includes three major components:

1. personal initiative;
2. therapy; and
3. a support group.

In addressing recovery from these different angles or directions, a total program is being structured and utilized. The idea of this particular three-part approach to recovery is to help a person understand how she/he can apply the principles of the Recovery Medicine Wheel as a complete program. Below is a diagram of the optimal recovery model.

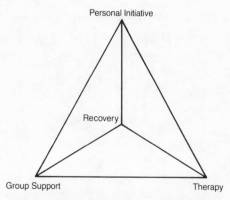

**THE OPTIMAL RECOVERY MODEL**

The benefits of applying the principles of the Recovery Medicine Wheel in such a manner are obvious. When a person uses the same step approach (the Recovery Medicine Wheel) in her or his personal thinking and reflecting, in groups and in therapy, it gives that approach strength and validity. In addition, confusion is reduced when groups, therapists and individuals operate under and reinforce the same principles. With this harmony among the component parts of the person's recovery program, good sustained progress in a positive direction is enhanced.

In the following pages you will find a detailed description of how each component of the optimal recovery model can become part of your recovery program. Of course, it can be helpful to use the Recovery Medicine Wheel in any one of these life and recovery areas (personal initiative, therapy, support groups). The message here is not that the optimal recovery model is an "all or nothing" approach. Rather, it suggests that you can maximize your potential for positive, strong, sustained recovery by applying the Recovery Medicine Wheel principles in the manner that is recommended by the optimal recovery model.

### Personal Initiative

Before beginning any program with hopes of success, a person must be committed to recovery. Just as the Recovery Medicine Wheel states, "Beginning today I will acknowledge that change in my life must begin with me." This statement clearly conveys the need for a recovering person to understand that she or he must honestly and sincerely desire recovery. In addition, that person also must be willing to work the steps of the Recovery Medicine Wheel, not just to please or quiet others, but to help him or herself. Without an honest desire to recover, no program, group or person will help.

Personal initiative must begin with a statement to the self, a statement such as, "I want to recover and I am willing to make the changes that will help me help myself." Following such a statement, that individual then needs to read and think about each step in the Recovery Medicine Wheel.

To do this effectively (especially at first), it helps to write down your thoughts. For example, if you read step one in the West (Beginning today I will speak honestly with myself), a number of things could come to mind. You may start by saying to yourself, "Alcohol makes me go out of control," and end up focusing on feelings such as, "I am always angry" or "I spend most of my time feeling depressed." Whatever the case, write those thoughts and feelings down. Putting things on paper can sometimes help you get intense emotions under control. *Having thoughts written down also serves to help you remember when it comes time to talk to a therapist or share in a group.*

## Therapy

The use of the Recovery Medicine Wheel in therapy can act to bring focus and direction to the therapeutic session. As the client reviews his or her progress on a certain step or in a particular life area, the therapist can provide objectivity, a clearer sense of reality and support. In addition, therapists also can help their recovering clients gain insight, as well as assist them in the recognition of thought or behavior patterns that might lead to relapse.

Because of the great potential therapy has for contributing positively to your overall recovery program, care should be taken in who is chosen to provide that service. Don't be afraid to shop around. When looking for a therapist who can help you in your construction of a total recovery program, look for the following qualities:

1. Knowledge of substance abuse, ACoA and co-dependent issues.
2. An understanding of the long-term effects of life in a dysfunctional family or system.
3. An open and non-judgmental attitude.
4. A willingness to work with you in the application of the Recovery Medicine Wheel principles in your recovery program.

In addition to these qualifications, look also for a therapist with whom you feel comfortable. Since recovering people often have a great deal of difficulty with trust issues, it will be important for you to locate a person with whom you feel you can be open and honest. Although it may take some work to locate a therapist who meets your needs, in the long run, you will find that your time and effort was well spent.

## The Recovery Support Group

The support group is an integral part of anyone's overall recovery program. Support groups provide participating members with a sense of belonging. In addition, when recovering people have the opportunity to share their problems, feelings and frustrations with others, the realization that they are not alone in their struggles is made clear. Finally, support groups help recovering individuals stay sober, straight, positive, health-oriented or whatever by providing just what the name implies—support. Therefore, participation in a recovery support group needs to be a part of every recovering person's program.

However, just going out and finding a Recovery Medicine Wheel support group is not that simple. At present, the Recovery Medicine Wheel approach is very new and only a handful of groups exist.

Nevertheless, this does not mean that you will have to do without. A support group formation process will be outlined in the following pages. Again, this requires work on your part. But just as locating a compatible therapist is time well spent, so is the formation of a Recovery Medicine Wheel support group.

### Forming Your Recovery Medicine Wheel Support Group

To begin, we will explore group membership and formation. In the initial stages, this task requires talking with other recovering persons to see if they are interested in forming a group. Although some people may react to the Recovery Medicine Wheel with disinterest or negativity, there are still plenty of people out there who are searching for something new, something more in recovery; it is those persons who will become the core from which your group can grow.

Keep in mind that the willingness of potential group members to work the steps of the Recovery Medicine Wheel is far more important than whether or not they are drug addicts, alcoholics, co-dependents or ACoAs. In fact, the mixing of different people within a single group can help each person understand that they have many issues, feelings and fears in common. In addition, mixed groups allow us to see addiction from another angle. ACoAs can learn what life is like for the person with the addiction. Chemically dependent people are afforded the opportunity of understanding what may have been experienced by their children. Co-dependent individuals will be better able to comprehend the roles they have played in dysfunctional marriages, relationships or family systems. In general, all involved can learn and benefit.

Nevertheless, if you feel you are not ready for a mixed group, for whatever reason, do not hesitate to form "pure" groups (exclusively ACoAs, co-dependents or chemically dependent persons). The only warning that should be given to "pure" groups is that they need to take care not to become "gripe groups." This means, don't spend all of your time complaining about others.

For example, ACoAs who focus only on what their parents did will have a hard time moving on in recovery. Yes, these feelings need to be brought out, but no, you do not need to get stuck in them. The same holds true for chemically addicted and co-dependent people. Recognize and acknowledge your feelings, your anger, your frustrations, but don't become paralyzed by them. Rather, learn to explore, express, experience, process, resolve and move on.

## Rules And Structure

Finally, we look at group rules and structure. How should the steps of the Recovery Medicine Wheel be addressed in a group setting? How should new members be familiarized with the group? What should the basic group rules be? All of these questions are valid and important when considering how to structure and operate a Recovery Medicine Wheel group. However, regardless of the original instructions with which they begin, each group will develop rules and procedures that fit their particular needs. Therefore, the suggestions for group structure stated in this section should be used only as a guide.

First, the manner in which the Recovery Medicine Wheel is constructed serves as a form of structure in and of itself. If a person is following the steps of the Recovery Medicine Wheel, he or she is already imposing some form of structure in his or her life. However, as was suggested earlier in this book, the Recovery Medicine Wheel seems to work best if individuals and groups start in either the West (the realm of introspective thought) or the North (the physical realm) and continue around the wheel in a sunwise or clockwise direction. The West or North are suggested starting points because each of these realms begins by looking at denial, addictive lifestyles and poor health habits. In addition, most people beginning recovery are not yet ready to address issues in the realm of knowledge and enlightenment (East) or within the spiritual realm of existence (South). Recovering people must begin at the level of recognizing and dealing with dysfunctional behavior and, although each realm of the Recovery Medicine Wheel has validity for persons at any stage of recovery, it will be best understood if the West or the North are used as beginning points. After choosing the realm within which you will begin walking the steps of the Recovery Medicine Wheel, complete each step in that realm before moving on to the next area of the wheel.

At the present time, some of the Recovery Medicine Wheel groups in existence are choosing to work on one step per group meeting. Other groups are reading through all the steps at every meeting and then choosing a single step for further discussion. The method your group chooses will be up to you to decide as members. Still, however, it should be noted that focusing on more than one step for discussion per group meeting can be confusing, especially at first. Therefore, wait until group members are familiar with the Recovery Medicine Wheel before choosing more than one step to work per session.

After a group has worked through all the steps of the Recovery Medicine Wheel, any number of formats can be chosen for further meetings. The group may decide to work the entire wheel again, open itself up to suggestions from members as to which step should be focused on in that session, vote on the step to be worked during each session, or even divide the group time spent on each step discussed so that competing interests of individual members can be accommodated. In fact, groups can even assign themselves a step to work on between sessions with the intent of having that step chosen as the focus of the next group meeting.

### For New Members

When new members express an interest in joining the group, they should first be asked to read the Recovery Medicine Wheel book. This will give them a more complete understanding of what the Recovery Medicine Wheel is all about. In addition, the group will not need to suspend its agenda each time someone joins just so that person can be oriented. When a new member joins an active, vital group, it won't be long before he or she can participate fully.

Lastly, group rules need to be discussed. Some groups may choose to be anonymous, calling each other by first name only and identifying themselves by first name only when speaking to the public. Other groups may not feel the need for anonymity, but instead may establish the rule that what is said in the group remains in the group. The stating of rules such as, "No violence or threats of violence" can be done, but is not really necessary since the Recovery Medicine Wheel already addresses this issue. In fact, as noted earlier, a great deal of group structure is inherent in the Recovery Medicine Wheel. Therefore, elaborate rules of conduct and interaction will not be needed if the steps are followed by each participating group member. The Recovery Medicine Wheel way, as experienced through the group, can be a powerful and positive part of anyone's recovery. Do not hesitate to involve yourself in a recovery group. The support you receive from others who, like you, are struggling with many of the same problems, can and will help you stay on the path of recovery.

# 5

# The Whole Human Path

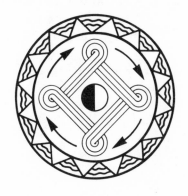

*"All of life is a sacred medicine wheel. The old songs, the old teachings and the old ways are all lessons for us; lessons that point us in the right direction. If we follow that sacred path the medicine wheel will always turn inside of us."*

Glen John/Navajo Medicine Man/Arizona, 1989.

To walk the steps of the Recovery Medicine Wheel is to follow a path that will lead us in the direction of becoming more fully human. I call this path the whole human path. Whereas addiction and addictive life patterns lead only to stagnation and death, the whole human path leads instead to continuous renewal throughout the natural course of our lifetime. Within the positive living way of the Recovery Medicine Wheel (the whole human path), we can and will come to understand the many facets of our existence. Our sexuality, need for humor, desires, emotions, prejudices, preferences, spiritual selves, limitations and potentials all can be experienced, processed and understood within the balanced living way of the whole human path.

The steps of the Recovery Medicine Wheel are the guides to healthy recovery, but living those steps is walking the whole human path. When I read and practice the steps of the Recovery Medicine Wheel, I bring the words to life. Like the story of Peach Tree, I learn to live in a healthy, balanced way—a way that allows me to be continuously renewed. The steps of the Recovery Medicine Wheel keep me on the whole human path, a path to real living.

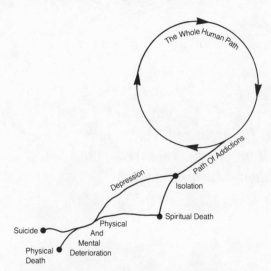

**THE WHOLE HUMAN PATH**

People who follow the whole human path will be those who begin to see the truth of addiction and addictive lifestyles. For example, many people in today's world see the use of chemical, mood-altering substances as a freeing experience, an expression of self, a personal choice or what have you. They see straight (non-using) people as repressed, lifeless; in short, no fun. However, these same people do not see where chemical substances become limiters of life. Drugs, including alcohol, are used to numb feelings, keep fear at bay, impart false self-confidence and a hundred other things. But in addition to this, chemical substance abuse also destroys bodies and brains and interferes with clear thinking. As people withdraw into the unbalanced state of addiction, their worlds become narrower and more focused on a single activity. In essence, they become increasingly limited.

A Pueblo Indian woman who had suffered for many years from addiction to alcohol explained very clearly what it meant for her to walk the whole human path. When she spoke of her recovery through the Recovery Medicine Wheel, she stated, "The Recovery Medicine Wheel feels right to me. It speaks to my heart. When I use the steps I feel like I am coming home to the teachings of the old ones, the grandfathers and grandmothers. When my body and my mind are not clouded anymore, I am free to see the mountains, to hear the river. I can laugh again. I know I am on the right path. I can see the world around me, and I am whole."

When it comes to addictive lifestyles, the thought processes become the culprit. Workaholism, religious fundamentalism, ideological fanaticism, etc. all act to limit a person's life. Whenever someone locks him or herself into a particular approach to living that discourages questioning, acquiring additional knowledge or seeking truth, that person is limited by addiction. Whether that addiction is to a president, a book, a guru, a lover or an idea, the net result is the same: Life becomes narrower, learning ceases, defenses are employed to protect beliefs, beliefs become truths, denial takes hold, the personality becomes rigid and the loving spirit dies. Therefore, whether manifested in chemical use, lifestyle or thought, the need to grow beyond addiction is clear. *Remember that addiction is a narrowing process while the living way of the whole human path is a broadening experience.*

Non-addicted or non-addictive people are those who can achieve a more complete freedom. A truer, deeper and more profound inner peace can be experienced when thinking is not clouded by chemicals, concepts or compulsive behaviors. When the fear of our own feelings is replaced by a desire to be fully human, addictive living can be seen for what it truly is: a hindrance, a limiter, a way of hiding from life. When this is understood, the idea of living a life free of addictions becomes appealing. It is no longer the way of giving up or of limiting the self. Rather, it becomes the way of growing, learning and living that has the potential of opening each of us up to millions of experiences, teachings and persons that would have never before been considered.

The Recovery Medicine Wheel provides the tools for us and the necessary steps that will lead us to and keep us on the whole human path. With its strong emphasis on balance, harmony, centeredness and freedom, the Recovery Medicine Wheel becomes not only a road to self-discovery, but a model for the maintenance of mind, body and spirit in a state of wellness. It is in seeking this state of well-being that we will be able to begin the process of setting aside our unsubstantiated fears, abandoning our rigid judgmental attitudes and opening ourselves to total learning. Through the Recovery Medicine Wheel, the living way of the whole human path is a reality, not just a dream or an ideal. So walk the steps. Grow to understand yourself and your world. Learn love and respect. Seek balance in living. As far as possible, make personal freedom real. Develop your spirituality. Explore, experience and enjoy life.

# 6

# Concluding

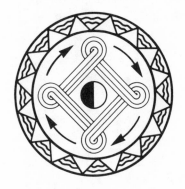

*"The message is out there for each of us to hear and it is as old as Mother Earth herself. If you listen with your heart, little by little, all of creation will begin to sing inside of you."*

*Anonymous Elder/Ojibwa/Ontario, Canada, 1986.*

Just as the first winds of spring carry the promise of
warmth to come, your own desire to recover brings with
it the promise of a fuller life. The Recovery Medicine
Wheel is a little book with big ideas. It is written to inspire
you, to let you know that change is possible. This book
has also been written to make you think, to cause you to
look at your beliefs, ideas, feelings and aspirations in life.

The Recovery Medicine Wheel is a gift, my gift to Native and natural people. In this book I have shared with
you what I have learned, what I know and what has
worked with me. It is my hope that through the Recovery
Medicine Wheel you will find your own sacred path to
recovery. So go forward; dare to dance in the sunlight.
The creation is alive around you; let yourself be alive
inside as well.

> *In the house of long life,*
> *there I wander.*
> *In the house of happiness,*
> *there I wander.*
> *Beauty before me,*
> *with it I wander.*
> *Beauty behind me,*
> *with it I wander.*
> *Beauty above me,*
> *with it I wander.*
> *Beauty below me,*
> *with it I wander.*
> *Beauty all around me,*
> *with it I wander.*
> *In old age traveling,*
> *with it I wander.*
> *On the beautiful trail I am,*
> *with it I wander.*
>
> *Navajo Prayer*

# Bibliography

Benton-Banai, **The Mishonis Book: The Voice of the Ojibwa.** Out of publication. Indian Country Press, 643 Virginia Street, St. Paul, Minnesota 55103, 1979.

Campbell, J. and Moyers, B. **The Power Of The Myth.** Doubleday, New York, 1988.

Easwaran, E. **God Makes The Rivers To Flow.** Nilgiri Press, Santa Cruz, 1982.

Fishel, R. **The Journey Within: A Spiritual Path To Recovery.** Health Communications, Pompano Beach, Florida, 1987.

Forrest, G. **How To Live With A Problem Drinker And Survive.** Atheneum Books, New York, 1985.

Kritsberg, W. **The Adult Children of Alcoholics Syndrome.** Health Communications, Pompano Beach, Florida, 1985.

Miller, A. **The Drama Of The Gifted Child.** Harper & Row, New York, 1983.

Peck, M.S. **People Of The Lie: The Hope For Healing Human Evil.** Simon & Schuster, New York, 1984.

Satir, V. **peoplemaking.** Science & Behavior Books, Palo Alto, 1972.

Schaef, A.W. **Co-dependence: Misdiagnosed And Mistreated.** Harper, 1986.

Storm, H. **Seven Arrows.** Ballantine Books, New York, 1972.

**Twelve Steps and Twelve Traditions.** Alcoholics Anonymous World Services, New York, 1952.

**Twenty-Four Hours A Day.** Hazelden, Center City, Minnesota, 1954.

Wallace, J. **Alcoholism: New Light On The Disease.** Edgehill, Newport, Rhode Island, 1985.

Wegscheider-Cruse, S. **Choicemaking: For Co-dependents, Adult Children and Spirituality Seekers.** Health Communications, Pompano Beach, Florida, 1985.

Whitfield, C.W. **A Gift To Myself.** Health Communications, Deerfield Beach, Florida, 1990.

Woititz, J.G. **Adult Children of Alcoholics.** Health Communications, Pompano Beach, Florida, 1983.

# Daily Affirmation Books from . . .
## Health Communications

*GENTLE REMINDERS FOR CO-DEPENDENTS: Daily Affirmations*
Mitzi Chandler

With insight and humor, Mitzi Chandler takes the co-dependent and the adult child through the year. Gentle Reminders is for those in recovery who seek to enjoy the miracle each day brings.

**ISBN 1-55874-020-1** $6.95

*TIME FOR JOY: Daily Affirmations*
Ruth Fishel

With quotations, thoughts and healing energizing affirmations these daily messages address the fears and imperfections of being human, guiding us through self-acceptance to a tangible peace and the place within where there is *time for joy.*

**ISBN 0-932194-82-6** $6.95

*AFFIRMATIONS FOR THE INNER CHILD*
Rokelle Lerner

This book contains powerful messages and helpful suggestions aimed at adults who have unfinished childhood issues. By reading it daily we can end the cycle of suffering and move from pain into recovery.

**ISBN 1-55874-045-6** $6.95

*DAILY AFFIRMATIONS: For Adult Children of Alcoholics*
Rokelle Lerner

Affirmations are a way to discover personal awareness, growth and spiritual potential, and self-regard. Reading this book gives us an opportunity to nurture ourselves, learn who we are and what we want to become.

**ISBN 0-932194-47-3**
**(Little Red Book)** $6.95
**(New Cover Edition)** $6.95

*SOOTHING MOMENTS: Daily Meditations For Fast-Track Living*
Bryan E. Robinson, Ph.D.

This is designed for those leading fast-paced and high-pressured lives who need time out each day to bring self-renewal, joy and serenity into their lives.

**ISBN 1-55874-075-9** $6.95

3201 S.W. 15th Street,
Deerfield Beach, FL 33442-8190
1-800-851-9100

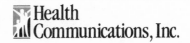 Health Communications, Inc.

# Other Books By . . .
# Health Communications

*ADULT CHILDREN OF ALCOHOLICS*
Janet Woititz

Over a year on *The New York Times* Best-Seller list, this book is the primer on Adult Children of Alcoholics.

**ISBN 0-932194-15-X**                    **$6.95**

*STRUGGLE FOR INTIMACY*
Janet Woititz

Another best-seller, this book gives insightful advice on learning to love more fully.

**ISBN 0-932194-25-7**                    **$6.95**

*BRADSHAW ON: THE FAMILY: A Revolutionary Way of Self-Discovery*
John Bradshaw

The host of the nationally televised series of the same name shows us how families can be healed and individuals can realize full potential.

**ISBN 0-932194-54-0**                    **$9.95**

*HEALING THE SHAME THAT BINDS YOU*
John Bradshaw

This important book shows how toxic shame is the core problem in our compulsions and offers new techniques of recovery vital to all of us.

**ISBN 0-932194-86-9**                    **$9.95**

*HEALING THE CHILD WITHIN: Discovery and Recovery for*
*Adult Children of Dysfunctional Families* — Charles Whitfield, M.D.

Dr. Whitfield defines, describes and discovers how we can reach our Child Within to heal and nurture our woundedness.

**ISBN 0-932194-40-0**                    **$8.95**

*A GIFT TO MYSELF: A Personal Guide To Healing My Child Within*
Charles L. Whitfield, M.D.

Dr. Whitfield provides practical guidelines and methods to work through the pain and confusion of being an Adult Child of a dysfunctional family.

**ISBN 1-55874-042-2**                    **$11.95**

*HEALING TOGETHER: A Guide To Intimacy And Recovery For*
*Co-dependent Couples* — Wayne Kritsberg, M.A.

This is a practical book that tells the reader why he or she gets into dysfunctional and painful relationships, and then gives a concrete course of action on how to move the relationship toward health.

**ISBN 1-55784-053-8**                    **$8.95**

3201 S.W. 15th Street,
Deerfield Beach, FL 33442-8190
1-800-851-9100

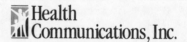
Health Communications, Inc.

# Books from . . .
# Health Communications

*PERFECT DAUGHTERS: Adult Daughters Of Alcoholics*
Robert Ackerman
Through a combined narrative of professional and anecdotal styles Robert
Ackerman helps restore a sense of balance in life for Adult Daughters of
Alcoholics.
**ISBN 1-55874-040-6**                                                    **$8.95**

*I DON'T WANT TO BE ALONE:*
*For Men And Women Who Want To Heal Addictive Relationships*
John Lee
John Lee describes the problems of co-dependent relationships and his
realization that he may be staying in such a relationship because of his
fear of being alone.
**ISBN 1-55874-065-1**                                                    **$8.95**

*SHAME AND GUILT: Masters Of Disguise*
Jane Middelton-Moz
The author uses myths and fairy tales to portray different shaming
environments and to show how shame can keep you from being the
person you were born to be.
**ISBN 1-55874-072-4**                                                    **$8.95**

*LIFESKILLS FOR ADULT CHILDREN*
Janet G. Woititz and Alan Garner
This book teaches you the interpersonal skills that can make your life easier
while improving your sense of self-worth. Examples are provided to help
clarify the lessons and exercises are given for practicing your new skills.
**ISBN 1-55874-070-8**                                                    **$8.95**

*THE MIRACLE OF RECOVERY:*
*Healing For Addicts, Adult Children And Co-dependents*
Sharon Wegscheider-Cruse
This is about the good news — that recovery from co-dependency is
possible. Sharon offers ways to embrace the positive aspects of one's
experience — to realize the strength that can come from adversity.
Celebrate your own miracle with this inspiring book.
**ISBN 1-55874-024-4**                                                    **$9.95**

SHIPPING/HANDLING: All orders shipped UPS unless weight exceeds 200 lbs., special routing is requested, or
delivery territory is outside continental U.S. Orders outside United States shipped either Air Parcel Post or Surface
Parcel Post. Shipping and handling charges apply to all orders shipped whether UPS, Book Rate, Library Rate, Air
or Surface Parcel Post or Common Carrier and will be charged as follows. Orders less than $25.00 in value add
$2.00 minimum. Orders from $25.00 to $50.00 in value (after discount) add $2.50 minimum. Orders greater than
$50.00 in value (after discount) add 6% of value. Orders greater than $25.00 outside United States add 15% of
value. We are not responsible for loss or damage unless material is shipped UPS. Allow 3-5 weeks after receipt of
order for delivery. Prices are subject to change without prior notice.

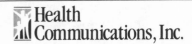

3201 S.W. 15th Street,
Deerfield Beach, FL 33442-8190
1-800-851-9100

**Health**
**Communications, Inc.**